My True-Life Story

of

Non-Hodgkin Lymphoma

Plus

Lower Leg Amputation

I0449340

By Trevor A Harris

ISBN: 978-1-365-68534-7

Introduction

This is the Story of my unexpected life experience and my journey of Non-Hodgkin T-Cell Lymphoma, which also resulted in the subsequent amputation of my left foot.

My name is Trevor Harris and I wrote this story in 2016, in plain language, as I remembered my painful and unwanted journey to hell and back many times, in the treatment of my Non-Hodgins T-Cell Lymphoma plus the Amputation of my left foot.

For privacy, in this story I have used first names only.

My intention in writing this story is to help others in understanding plus try and help make sense of this disease and in coping with Lymphoma plus Amputation.

More on these plus my thank you to all the people who have helped compile and edit this book can be found in the Appendix.

I dedicate this story to my Mother whom died of cancer, in 2002, at the age 86, and my Father, whom died in July 2009 at the age 93; and to all those people whom have suffered with Lymphoma and amputation.

Table of Contents

This Story begins in Late March 2014 when my life was changed forever.

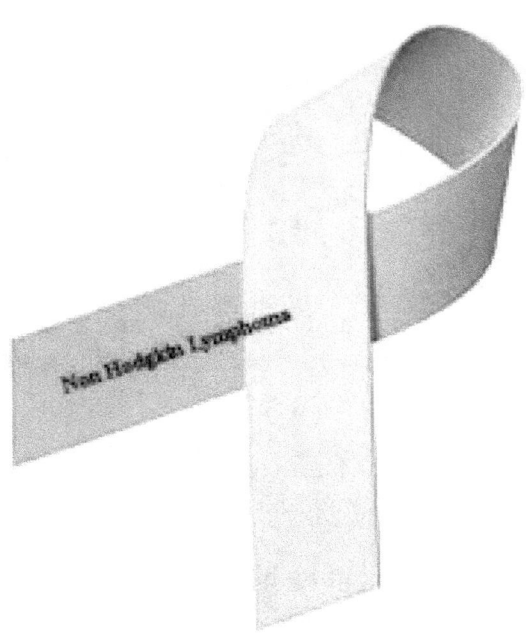

Chapter 1

Brinkworth, South Australia: March 2014

In late March 2014, I was I was fit and well and living in my caravan at Brinkworth having been touring around parts of Australia. *(refer to Appendix B: About myself)*

On the 21st March 2014, due to having a bad cough, I had made an appointment with my Doctor at the Virginia Medical Centre, Virginia; a 45-minute drive. He prescribed antibiotics 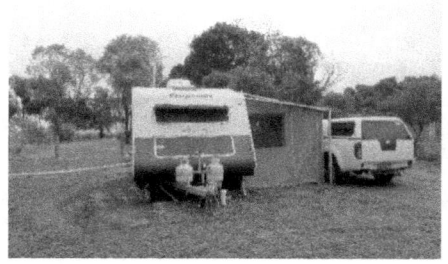 for my chest cough, and I also had an inoculation for influenza, plus I gave a blood sample to test my Cholesterol level.

Then around the 26th March 2014, I became sick at home, in my caravan at Brinkworth.

I was coughing plus getting high temperatures having hot sweaty spells just drenching the bed plus cold shivering spells; also, vomiting and my whole body shaking violently for an hour at a time, plus I had swollen feet.

Yes, I was stubborn thinking it would all go away, as I had an appointment with my Doctor in Virginia for Friday

28th March, and I was putting off going to the Doctor beforehand.

On Friday, 28 March 2014 I was due to go to the doctor for the results of the blood tests but, I found I was too sick to drive there. I rang my doctor in Virginia and explained all my symptoms and he considered that I was very sick, and he called an ambulance for me.

A few minutes later, I received a phone call asking for me to confirm that I required an ambulance, which I did. On Friday, 28 March 2014 around 11:30am, a local Paramedic arrived at my Home/Caravan.

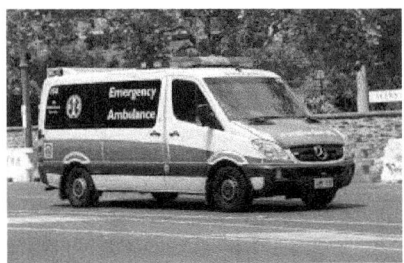

Handily, the female Paramedic only lived a few houses along the road. She came fully equipped, as the ambulance was coming from Snowtown, a small town about 15 minutes further afield. Soon another local cadet arrived and the ambulance arrived shortly after.

Firstly, they checked me out and found my Oxygen level to be only 80% of what it should be, so they gave me Oxygen and stabilized me before transferring me to the ambulance.

Then they drove to Clare Hospital, South Australia, a 30-minute drive, where I was admitted

Chapter 2

Clare Hospital, South Australia, March 2014

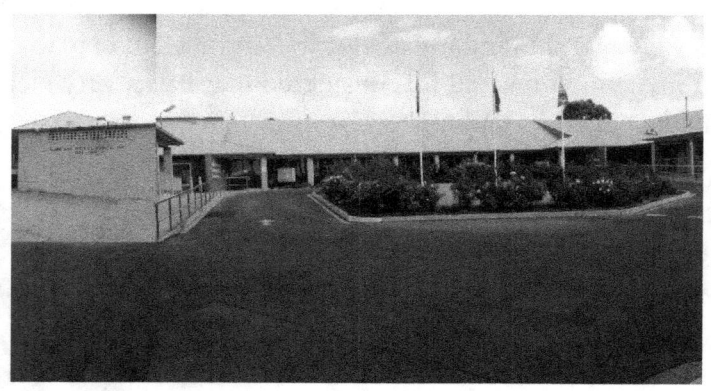

Clare Hospital provides a comprehensive range of medical and surgical services to patients from Clare and surrounding communities including the Lower and Mid North areas

I arrived at the Clare Hospital, by ambulance on Friday 28 March, 2014, at 12:45pm. They assessed me in Emergency. and then admitted me to a ward, awaiting. The Clare Hospital is quite modern, and I a two-person room with its own toilet and shower facilities etc.

There are no Resident Doctors at the Hospital, as they draw on Doctors from the local Medical Surgeries on a roster basis. The Doctors normally do their rounds in the evenings, after their daily practice duties.

The doctor from the Clare Medical Centre arrived at the hospital and advised it was just a chest problem, and that he would prescribe me more antibiotics. (As my previous doctor in Virginia had done) He also ordered a Chest X-ray.

28 March, 2014, I had a Chest X-ray and I was connected to a machine to monitor my heart.

The following day, 29 March, around 7:30pm, the same Doctor arrived on his rounds, and advised me that I needed to drink plenty of water, and to give the antibiotics time to work. At this time, I was feeling really tired and unwell.

Overnight I had two bed changes due to sweating profusely but awoke on the morning of 30 March feeling much better. The following night I had a better night awaking on the morning of 31 March feeling much better but far from okay.

The morning of 31 March I was told that the doctor had advised the hospital to discharge me, advising I was to continue taking my antibiotics. The hospital advised me they would be discharging me at 11am, as they expected the antibiotics to work. but I was to go to a doctor if I wasn't feeling better.

31 March 2014 Discharged from Clare Hospital
Back in Brinkworth

On 1 April 2014 I was back home in my Caravan in Brinkworth, where I had had several overnight sweats, soaking all my bedding. My temperature seemed to have come down and the swelling in my feet had gone down a little bit.

Tuesday, 1st April I went to town and I purchased an Electronic Thermometer and Blood pressure machine, similar to what they used in the hospital, so that I could keep track of my own temperature and blood pressure.

My temperature at this stage was 38° C and the normal is 36° C. The weather at the time was really hot, close to 40°C so it was really rather difficult to judge my condition with the outside temperature being so high, but I did have air conditioning going on high.

I checked my blood pressure regularly which was fine.

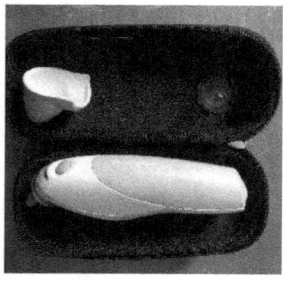 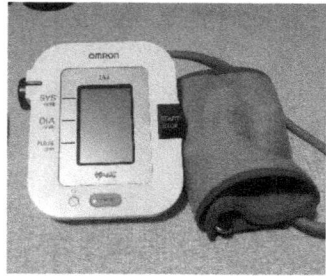

Thermometer   Blood Pressure machine

By Thursday, 3 April, I was still feeling unwell. Both my feet were swollen, and I was still using the antibiotics.

On Friday 4th April I thought I had an appointment with the doctor, but didn't realize till after driving to the doctors in Clare that it was for Monday. I was still feeling unwell and my feet were still swollen. I was advised to go to the Clare Hospital on the Monday, 7 April at 9am.

I went to the Clare hospital at 9 am on the Monday, however, the doctor had forgotten to organize the appointment.

On the morning of 8 April I was very sick, and so I went to see a doctor at the Clare Medical Centre. The doctor was not the first doctor who had previously attended me at the Clare Hospital. This Doctor was listed as the Registrar at the Medical Centre, and I spent a long time at the surgery (costing me well over $100). He turned to me and said I want you to go straight to the hospital now. This was around midday, and I explained that I had driven myself there, and that I was not actually prepared for hospital. I needed to go home and gather some things together, so he said to do that and he would ring me later.

Later in the day he called and advised me to meet him at the Clare Hospital at 7pm to be readmitted.

8 April 2014 Readmitted to Clare Hospital

I was finally readmitted to the Clare Hospital at 9pm on the 8 April and was put on a drip. The nurse said to me I should have been admitted days before. Yes, as it happened, I had been admitted days before and then discharged. During the day I had Chest X-ray.

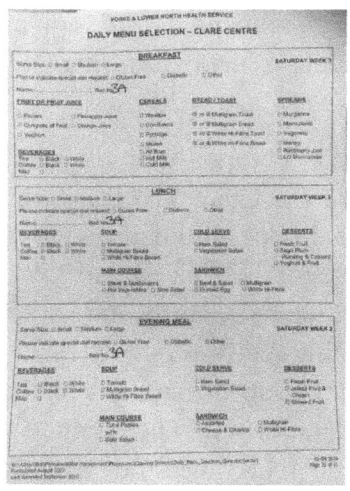

Above is a typical daily food menu served by the hospital

On the evening 9 April at the Clare Hospital the doctor did his rounds around 9pm, when "luckily" he saw at first hand my condition. I was shaking and sweating etc. He explained that he did not know what was wrong with me, and was concerned. He then advised me he had contacted the Lyell McEwin Hospital (in Adelaide) and advised them that he considered I had a stomach infection; I had been on antibiotic medication and that he was sending me to Lyell McEwin Hospital for specialist care.

Whilst standing beside my bed, he rang for an ambulance and he was asked if he wanted a helicopter or road ambulance, and chose the latter due to the cost of the helicopter.

I was then prepared for the transfer, and remember, as the ambulance was ready to leave, the nurse who had been caring for me, very kindly brought me a bottle of water. I also remember as the nurse walked back towards the door she appeared upset and crying; I feel she sensed I was very sick.

The ambulance left the Clare Hospital at 10:30pm and I was advised that the Ambulance was only able to go halfway, as they have certain areas they work within. I would be changing into a second Ambulance at Tarlee.

Arriving at Tarlee, after a one-hour drive, I still felt okay and I asked to go to the toilet, after which I was then transferred into the second ambulance which was waiting to take me on to the second part of the journey, Another one-hour drive to the Lyell McEwin Hospital in Adelaide. The trip went well and luckily, I was feeling okay whilst being transported.

Upon arriving at 12:30am, 10 April 2014, I was transferred into the Emergency Department of the Lyell McEwin Hospital.

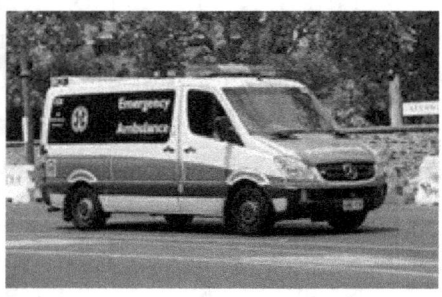

Similar Ambulance that transported me from Clare Hospital to Lyell McEwin Hospital.

Summary of Electronic Tests

28 March 2014: Heart Monitor

28 March 2014: X-ray of Chest

9 April 2014: X-ray of Chest

Chapter 3

Lyell McEwin Hospital

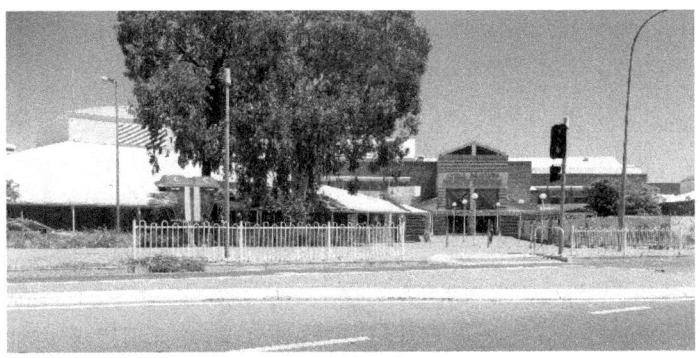

The Lyell McEwin Hospital is a 385-bed acute care teaching hospital located in Adelaide, South Australia that provides a full range of medical, surgical, diagnostic, emergency and support services to a population of more than 300,000 people living primarily in Adelaide's northern suburbs and nearby towns

The ambulance arrived at the Lyell McEwin Hospital at 12.30am, on the 10 April, 2014, where I was taken immediately to the Emergency Department.

The Emergency Department was very busy, as they were short staffed, and had little time to spend with me other than check my vital signs (temperature, blood pressure etc.). They attached leads and a heart monitor to my chest, and then left me alone in the holding area, as they needed to attend to other patients.

About 5am I started feeling sick again. Besides the chills and the sweats, I had the rigors (rigors is where the body shakes all over uncontrollably). As I was in the middle of a temporary/holding area, I had no emergency or attention button, and was quite distressed.

Someone walked past, so I yelled out, and put up my arm drawing attention to myself. Next thing I was surrounded by two doctors and three nurses, talk about attention, but I was not putting on a show.

One doctor came beside me, and said to me, looking into my eyes, "Mr. Harris you are very, very sick!" I was thinking yes I am. Then he said, "I need your help, I want you to do this......". I cannot remember exactly what he said, but it was something to help stop the shaking. I believe they gave me an injection and also some pills, but I am not sure. Within half an hour or so I was feeling better again, and more settled.

They then shifted me, still within the Emergency Department, into my own cubicle. Meanwhile, I sent a text to my son asking if he could come to the hospital.

At this time a young female doctor, who was situated in the middle hub of the Emergency Department, came out to me and asked me questions about my medical history. She must have returned about ten times, asking me different questions. She was thorough compiling my past medical history, so they could get a full picture of my situation. Everything was quite professional, and I was very impressed.

My son arrived, and it was good to see him. I was feeling alright at this stage, but it had been a very long night and I was very tired.

I was later transferred to a newly built ward where I had my own private room complete with all facilities, including a large recliner-style chair and some nice large windows with the sun streaming in.

On the 11 April at 9 am a Consultant Physician, of many years of experience, arrived to check me over. He was accompanied by six student doctors, as all the hospitals in Adelaide are known as learning hospitals. Throughout my admissions in the chain of five hospitals, at most times, there were student doctors in attendance.

The Physician asked the student doctors what they felt was wrong with me. They all had my medical history that had been recorded earlier, so they had had time to analyze my past history and my present symptoms, however none of them could come up with a correct diagnosis.

The Physician then asked me to lift my right arm, going directly to my armpit and feeling the lymph glands. Looking up to his students he stated one word, "swollen", then lent across me and felt the lymph glands under my left armpit. Again, he turned to the students and said "swollen".

He then asked me if it was okay for each of the students to feel under my armpits. I said 'yes', so each in turn came and felt the swollen lymph glands under my armpits.

The doctor then proceeded to undertake a normal examination, as he already had all the vital signs and other tests in my records. I was then programed for a CT scan later that day.

I underwent a full body CT scan 11 April, 2014

During the day, I regularly had more blood tests, as well as regular blood pressure, temperature readings, etc. I was advised that they were going to have to operate underneath my right armpit to remove two of my lymph glands. This operation was carried out late in the day on the 15 April.

On the 16 April, the Surgeon consulted with me, advising that we would have to wait some days for the results of the biopsy of the Lymph Node glands, which had been removed.

At this stage, it was around the Anzac Day Holiday, plus the long weekend following. A decision was made to release me from hospital whilst they waited for the results of the CT scan and the biopsy of the Lymph Node glands.

Later on Wednesday, 16 April I was discharged from the Lyell McEwin Hospital.

As I was not well enough to return to my caravan in Brinkworth my son and daughter, (whom had recently arrived from New Zealand), arranged for me to stay in a motel, reasonably close to the hospital,

After a couple of days at the motel, on the night of the 19 April, I was still getting chills, sweating and shaking very badly. This was happening up to three times in one night, making the whole bed soaking wet.

On the morning of the 20 April I rang my son who was at work, and explained how sick I was, and we decided I should go straight back to the Lyell McEwin Hospital.

On 20 April, I arrived back at the Lyell McEwin Hospital, where they advised that they had the results of the CT scan as well as the results of the biopsy from the lymph glands. The conclusion was that I had Non-Hodgkin's T-Cell Lymphoma.

Once again, I was connected to the heart monitor; had another chest X-ray plus a CT scan, and an Ultra sound of my abdomen.

At this stage I was still very sick with swollen and very sore feet. About 1am, that night, I wanted to get out of bed into the large recliner chair nearby to try and relieve the pain in my left foot. I pushed the 'Attention' button to call the nurse whom subsequently came to help me get into the chair. For some reason, she did not appear happy about assisting me move from my bed into the chair.

After I was settled, and she was about to leave, I asked her what was her problem. She advised I was very 'demanding', it wasn't the answer that I expected from a nurse.

This was the only time in the many months in hospital that I was treated adversely by anyone in the hospital system.

I had advised the nursing staff of my sore feet, but no attention seemed to be given to my feet, and it seems they were only interested in my other symptoms regarding the cancer.

Then on the 22April I was advised that I was immediately being transferred to Queen Elizabeth Hospital, and that day around 4pm

Transferred to the Queen Elizabeth Hospital by ambulance and admitted to the Haematology Ward.

Summary of Electronic Tests and Operations:
10 April 2014: Attached to Heart monitor

11 April 2014: CT scan of whole body.

15 April 2014: Biopsy of Armpit Glands.

20 April 2014: Attached to Heart monitor

20 April 2014: Ultra sound of abdomen

20 April 2014: X-ray of Chest

20 April 2014: CT scan of whole body.

Chapter 4

Queen Elizabeth Hospital - Part One
Arrival 22 April 2014

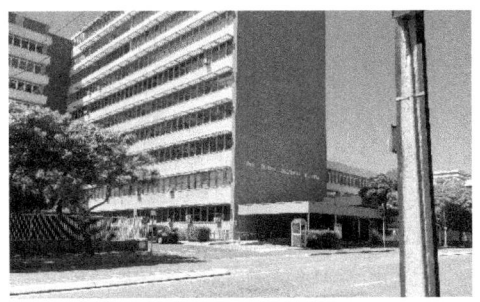

The Queen Elizabeth Hospital is a 311 bed, Acute Care teaching hospital that provides inpatient, Outpatient, Emergency and Mental Health Services to a population of more than 250,000 people living primarily in Adelaide's Western Suburbs

Around 4pm, on Tuesday 22 April, 2014, I was transferred by ambulance from the Lyell McEwin Hospital at Elizabeth, to the Queen Elizabeth Hospital, Woodville, in the Western Suburbs of Adelaide.

Upon arrival I was admitted to the Haematology/Oncology Ward (a newly built ward) and given a private room, with all amenities including a fridge, and large windows from which I could watch the movement of people and cars in the street outside.

The nursing staff were very welcoming, and very helpful. At this stage I was feeling fine, but I did have swollen feet. My left foot in particular, was very sore, and the staff advised me that they needed to speak to my son. This was in the evening, so I asked him to try and get to the ward before half past seven, which he did, and I believe he spoke to the Doctor.

Unbeknownst to me, my condition of Lymphoma was not good at this time. About a year later the Oncology Doctor advised me that he had not expected me to live, and that he had prescribed a treatment that he would normally only prescribe a 21-year-old with the stamina to survive.

The hospital gave me medication, and I am unsure what it was, but I suspect it was steroids. I awoke on Wednesday, 23 April, after a good night with no symptoms, other than my left foot being very sore.

They were desperately wanting to start my Chemotherapy treatment for my Lymphoma, it was necessary to sort the problems with my foot first.

I was advised that I could have pain relief for the foot, and during the day I was taken to have another CT Scan. Then around 5pm I was taken to Radiology, and had my left foot X-rayed.

As they couldn't find anyone to take me back to the ward I was stuck down in X-Ray for a few hours. It wasn't really a problem because I was in the Ward all day, and it was good to be out of it for a little while. It was a big day, and I was completely stuffed at the end of it, to put it mildly.

I was attached to a heart monitoring machine for a few days and I believe all was well in that area.

Each day, apart from the incredibly caring nursing staff, I was visited by various hospital professionals including Specialist Doctors, Social workers, Clinical Psychologist and Physiotherapists.

Whilst in hospital, and over the following year, I was visited, and had appointments with Sara, my Clinical Psychologist. She guided me through all the uncharted waters of having Cancer, plus the trauma of having my foot amputated. Please refer to the Appendix for the Psychologist Reports.

I was advised that the following day, Thursday, 24th April, I would be going to the Royal Adelaide Hospital to have a PET Scan. Rather than go in an ambulance my son said he could take me, which the hospital allowed.

My appointment was for approximately midday, on Thursday, 24 April.

Chapter 5

Royal Adelaide Hospital

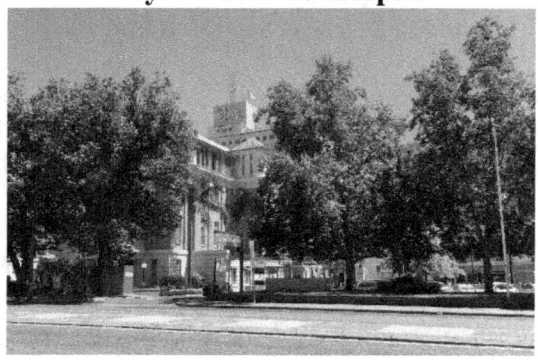

The Royal Adelaide Hospital (RAH),is Adelaide's (and South Australia's) largest hospital. With 800 beds, the RAH provides tertiary health care services for South Australia and provides secondary care clinical services to residents of Adelaide's City Centre and inner suburbs

On the morning of 24 April at 11:30am my son picked me up from the Haematology Ward at the Queen Elizabeth Hospital, and we drove to the Royal Adelaide Hospital. He took me, by hospital wheelchair, due to my sore foot, up to the Department of Nuclear medicine to undergo a PET Scan.

The PET Scan machine basically takes a 3D image of the whole of your body by using the radioactive material they had injected in my blood.

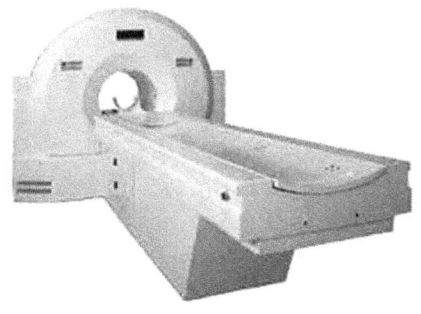

The photo above is typical of a PET Scan machine

There are special preparations before a PET Scan as follows; a patient is required to fast from food for six (6) hours prior to the study.

It is also important to be well hydrated, so drinking plenty of water is encouraged. You will also need to abstain from any strenuous exercise for twelve (12 hours) prior to the scan, as this may affect the distribution of glucose within the body.

[The PET Scan procedure is as follows;
A drip line is inserted into a vein in the arm. Then a small amount of blood will be taken through this to test the blood sugar level.

A saline drip is then connected to the line to ensure hydration. After the drip is inserted the patient will need to lie down in a quiet room for at least 15 minutes beforehand, and an hour after the administration of the tracer.

The patient is be given two drinks of oral contrast; the taste is not unpleasant. One is drunk when the patient is first taken to the resting room, and the other just prior to the scan. These drinks ensure that the bowel is visible on the images, thereby assisting in the analysis.

A doctor will then administer the tracer via the drip. The tracer is a small amount of radioactive glucose, which will not cause any side effects.

The PET/CT scan begins approximately 60-90 minutes after the injection. During the scan, the patient lies on the scanning bed, which moves through the PET/CT scanner. The scan will take approximately 40 minutes. The radioactive glucose releases positrons, which are detected by the scanner and displayed as images.]

The hour following was very long, being in a very small dark room, but I guess that was the least of my worries.

At the end of the hour I was taken into another room and placed on the bed of the PET Scan, machine which looks very similar to a CT Scan machine. I had to lay perfectly still for 45 minutes, with some difficulty, whilst the PET Scan machine carried out the scan.

I kept my iPhone constantly beside and at the completion of the PET Scan I contacted my son, whom came and picked me up, and returned me to the Queen Elizabeth Hospital.

I was very hungry as I had been fasting for the PET Scan so we stopped and bought some pies. Then we made a detour, where I bought myself a brand-new wheelchair. I am not even sure of what prompted me to do this, but it did turn out to become very necessary.

Unfortunately, the results of the PET Scan confirmed the seriousness of my Non-Hodgkin's T-Cell Lymphoma, as shown in the following images.

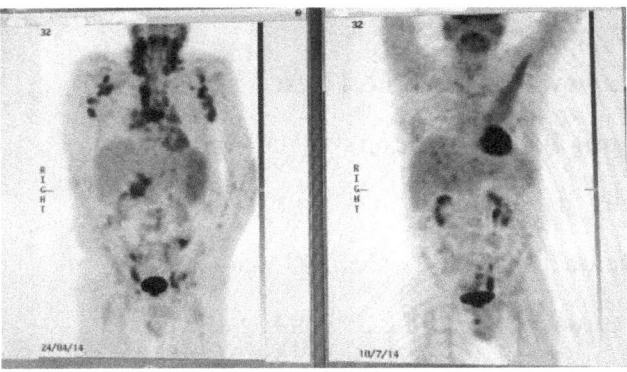

These are my PET Scan images: "Positron Emission Tomography "

A PET scan uses radiation to create three dimensional, colour images of the functional processes in the human body.

The image on the left above, is from my first PET Scan, on 24 April, 2014, and the one on the right from my PET Scan on 10 July, 2014 after six rounds of Chemotherapy.

The Cancer is all the small black objects known as Cancer hot spots (like dots) on the left scan, the larger black objects are organs. The scan on the right, done after Chemotherapy, shows no Cancer.

I returned to the Royal Adelaide Hospital for a PET Scan on three more occasions, having a total of four PET Scans over my treatment period.

Summary of Electronic Tests:

24 April 2014: PET Scan #1 whole body

10 July 2014: PET Scan #2 whole body

08 October 2014: PET Scan #3 whole body

09 February 2015: PET Scan #4 whole body

Chapter Six

Queen Elizabeth Hospital - Part Two
Returned from the Royal Adelaide Hospital

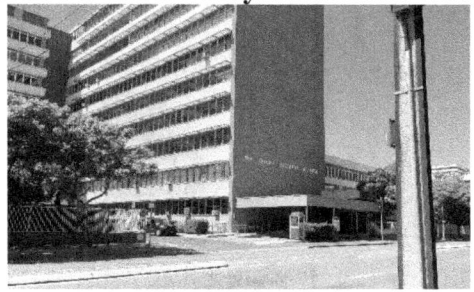

I arrived back at the Queen Elizabeth Hospital from the Royal Adelaide Hospital, on Thursday, 24 April 2014 at 3.30pm, and was advised by staff, that they desperately wanted to commence the Chemotherapy treatment for my Lymphoma.

When the doctors came on their daily round, Doctor Julia, a female Oncologist, noticed my swollen feet out of the end of the bed. She must have observed that one of my feet did not look right, as she kept poking her finger on the flesh, finding that the blood was not returning to the left foot.

Doctor Julia concluded there was a problem with my blood flow in the left leg, so the Chemotherapy had to be postponed, as firstly they needed to sort out the problems with my left foot.

I was taken for an ultrasound scan on my left foot at 6:30pm, and was advised the ultrasound showed that my foot was not looking good.

Then I was advised that they were going to operate that evening, at the top of my left thigh to check the blood flow in my left leg, as they suspected there could be a blockage in the main artery.

As I had been out most of the day, and arrived back very hungry due to fasting for the PET Scan, I indulged in a good meal. As a result, I complicated the situation, and they needed to wait a further six hours before operating. It was after midnight when they finally operated.

The reason for the Amputation was due to a lack of blood flow to the left foot. This may well have been due to the Lymphoma but has never been confirmed. The only explanations are in the reports by the Surgeon in the Appendix section.

The following is a diary of the days after the operation on my left thigh, and the results which affected my further treatment for Lymphoma, and the amputation of my foot.

On April 25, the Vascular Surgeon came to see me in the morning and advised that he had found a blockage in my leg. He explained the blockage was a white substance which they had managed to clear, and were now waiting to see if the blood flow to the foot returned. I cannot remember much about the rest of the day but they must have visited me later that evening.

The Surgeon advised me that the blood flow had not returned and suggested that they could open up my calf muscle to see if they could clear out any blockages. The Surgeon then explained that he wasn't confident that they could repair the blood flow, and that the next procedure would have to be to amputation of my left foot, due to the length of time the foot had been deprived of blood flow.

I agreed to allow them to operate on the calf muscle, understanding if it was not successful they would have to amputate my foot. To complicate things yet again, I had recently eaten and they were forced to operate for a second night in a row, in the early hours of the morning.

On April 26, at 6:30am I desperately needed to go to the toilet, and there was no nurse around. I hopped out of bed to walk to the toilet and when I put my left foot on the floor, there was an excruciating pain. I crashed to the floor as I was in so much pain, and I could not hold my bladder. I wet all over the floor, and as I couldn't reach my buzzer I yelled out, and the nurse came running.

It was very embarrassing, but as far as the nurse was concerned there was nothing to be embarrassed about, and it was all part of the job for her. Then she lifted me up, how I am not sure, and helped me to the toilet, and then cleaned up after me. I had a shower using the shower chair on wheels as a wheelchair.

Later that morning the Vascular Surgeon came to visit me and advised that the operation from the night before was unsuccessful. This meant that they urgently needed to amputate my left foot as if it was not done it may lead to the amputation of my whole left leg.

I agreed to the operation on April 27, which was yet again, carried out late at night being the third nightly operation I had had in a row.

Early the next morning, on April 28, the Surgeon came to check on me and advised that the amputation had been successful.

I was now in the High Dependency Unit, known as "HDU" where the nurse is present at the bedside at all times (24/7) and is not allowed to leave until relieved by another nurse.

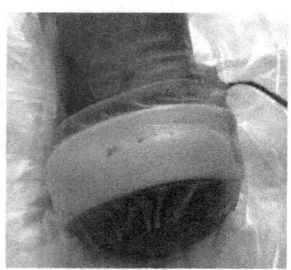

Stump after operation with protection

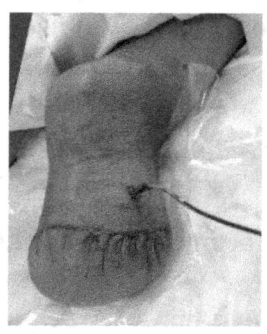

Stump after operation without protection

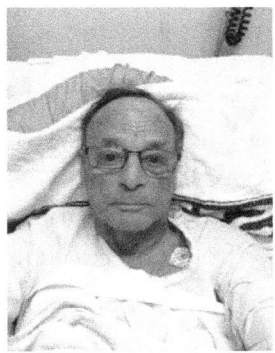 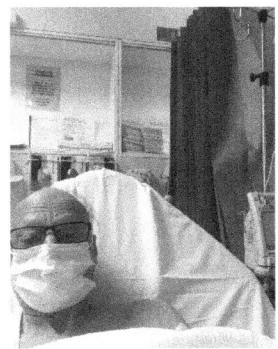

Myself in the High Dependency Unit (HDU)

At 8am on Monday, 28 April, the Surgical Team visited me after the operation, however, the following few days were a blank as I was heavily sedated.

At this time, I didn't know a lot about what was going on around me. I was in the HDU, but had no idea what went on during the day or night. I seemed to be awake during the night and asleep during the day. I remember the nurse was at my bedside 24/7, and they used torches at night; it was quite eerie with the place being in darkness. The nurses seemed to be taking my blood pressure and temperature every hour.

In the mornings, the nurse gave me a wash in bed, as at that stage I was not up and about at all. My son and daughter would come and visit me, but I was always asleep. One time that my Daughter visited I declared I just wanted to end it all as I was just so sick, this was the only time in my journey that this happened.

During the night, I had more sweats and chills, which were signs of the Lymphoma. The Oncology Department wanted to commence the Chemotherapy, but had to delay the treatment, the reason being that when you have Chemo it nulls your immune system and thus you have no healing properties and so the Chemotherapy treatment could not start until I had healed sufficiently from my amputation.

They then moved me within the HDU, to a quieter area, as I was still sleeping for hours and hours due to the drugs and I remember the head nurse came to my bed and she sat on the floor, as my head was hanging over the side of the bed, while I was asking her why I was so drugged, the nurse was being very caring and explaining that it was necessary till I got over the operation.

By Sunday, 4 May, I was feeling better, and I was asked to do some exercises.

On Monday, 5 May I had a good night with no sweats or chills and I was moved from the HDU to the Cancer Ward. Here I had an operation to install a PICC line which would enable the Chemotherapy bottle to be connected.

The people from St Margaret Rehabilitation Hospital where I was to be relocated in the future, also came to explain the shift to rehabilitation.

Following yet another night of huge sweats on Tuesday, 6 May, the nurse again remade my bed. My temperature ranged each day, from 36.6C in the mornings to 40-44C in the evenings. Whenever my temperature went to 40C or above, the nurses were required to call a doctor, and a doctor was called most evenings.

They would give me Panadol to bring down my temperature, but I believed it was only causing the sweats. Later I found out that the Panadol was just a mask, (creating a false temp reading) and that my temperature came down by itself, without the medication and the doctor had advised that I could decline the Panadol, which I did.

My first round of Chemotherapy treatment commenced on Tuesday, 6 May, 2014. I was taken by wheelchair, from the Cancer Ward, to the Cancer Clinic on the floor above, where the Chemotherapy medication treatment was commenced.

This area had many large, comfortable chairs for the undertaking of the procedure. Firstly, they explained the process, following which they gave me some medication. Then I had to wait for approximately an hour, when they gave me a small waist type bag to hold the Chemotherapy bottle.

The small Chemotherapy bottle was placed in the bag, which had a pipe connecting it into the PICC Line in my arm. The staff explained I would be wearing this for four days. This is the period taken for the Chemotherapy solution to automatically inject into my blood flow. I then, at that time, had to take several Chemotherapy pills daily, for the next four days.

The Hospital Pharmacist came and explained my medication; what each pill/tablet did and the amount and frequency of each. This was about twenty (20) pills per day, as the attached sheet following.

Full details of my Chemotherapy Treatment are in the Chemotherapy Chapter refer to the Index.

MEDICATION LIST

Government of South Australia

Name: Trevor HARRIS D.O.B 3/9/1969 U.R.N. 830746
Allergies: Nil known Date 11/07/2014

Prepared by Pharmacy Department
The Queen Elizabeth Hospital
28 Woodville Road
Woodville South, SA 5011
Hospital Switchboard: 8222 6000
Pharmacy Department: 8222 6648

MEDICATION NAME AND STRENGTH	BRAND NAME(S)	WHAT THE DRUG IS USED FOR	RECOMMENDED DOSING SCHEDULE			
			Brkfst 7-8am	Lunch 11-1pm	Dinner 4-6pm	Bed 8-10pm
ASPIRIN Tablets 100mg	Cardiprin, Astrix, Spren.	To prevent the formation of blood clots	**1**			
PREGABALIN Capsules 25mg	Lyrica	For the treatment of neuropathic (nerve) pain	**2**			**2**
PANTOPRAZOLE Tablets 40mg *Swallow whole. Do not crush or chew*	Panto, Pantofast, Salpraz, Somac, Torzole, plus other brands.	To reduce acid levels in the stomach	**1**			**1**
FLUCONAZOLE Capsules 200mg	Diflucan, Dizole, Fluzole, Ozole, plus other brands	To treat and prevent fungal infections.	**1**			
FAMCICLOVIR 250mg	Ezovir, Famlo, Famvir, Favic, plus other brands	An antiviral medication	**2**			**2**
TRIMETHOPRIM with SULFAMETHOXAZOLE Tablets 160/800mg	Bactrim DS, Resprim Forte, Septrim Forte	This is an antibiotic – the entire course should be completed	Take ONE tablet TWICE a day on MONDAYS and THURSDAYS only			

The following medications are to be taken only when required

OXYCODONE Tablets 5mg	Endone	For the treatment of moderate to severe pain	Take ONE tablet up to FOUR times a day if required

The following medications are used to help you in your cancer journey

PREDNISOLONE Tablets 25mg AND 5mg Take these tablets with food to prevent stomach upset	Panafcortelone, Solone, Panafcort, Sone	Steroid medication as part of your chemotherapy treatment	Take FOUR 25mg tablets and TWO 5mg tablets (110mg total) each morning for FIVE days each chemo cycle (8/8/14-12/8/14)			
ETOPOSIDE capsules 100mg AND 50mg	Vepesid	Part of your chemotherapy treatment Take for FOUR days then STOP (8/8/14-11/8/14)	Brkfst 7-8am **1 x 100 mg & 1 x 50 mg**	Lunch 11-1pm	Dinner 4-6pm	Bed 8-10pm **1 x 100 mg**

Page 1 of 1 Profile prepared for Mr Trevor HARRIS; Unit Record Number 830746; by Dale Thompson, (Pharmacist), on 11/07/2014. Signed _____

My daily Medication List supplied by the Pharmacist

(A little bewildering for someone who hates taking any medication).

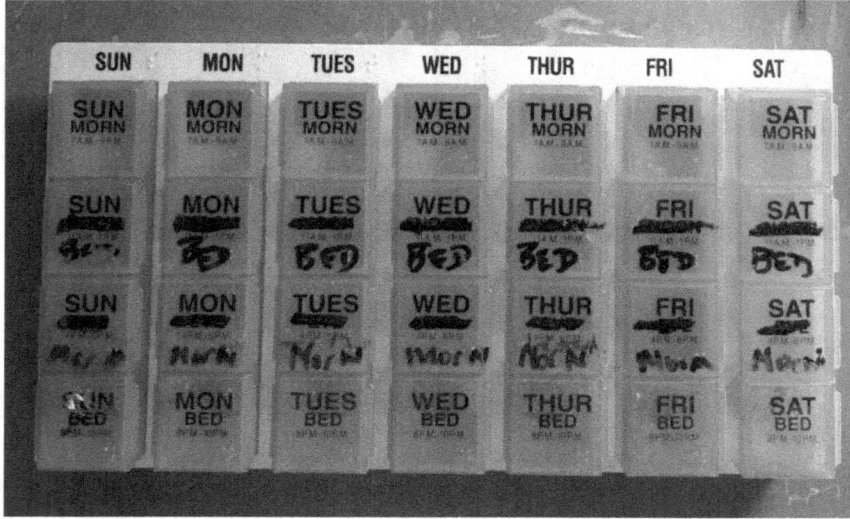

The pill box I used to control myself taking the pills

During the night, I had the sweats again, and the nurse changed my bed four times. I believe they then put me on some steroids, which appeared to stop the sweats and chills.

At 6:45am on Wednesday, 7 May, I was advised that I had a big day ahead of me. I had a good night with no sweats or chills, and slept all night.

My bottle of Chemotherapy finished on May 10, and it was removed. I was given an injection in the stomach which activated the Chemotherapy.

My Son Kevin had a meeting with the Oncologists and the rehabilitation hospital personnel, on Sunday, 11 May,

By Tuesday, 13 May I had had a catheter in for several days and it had become blocked. Although it was very uncomfortable, I was told that they could not remove the catheter until midnight. I was not sure why, but midnight came and went, and they did not remove the catheter until around 1am.

After a reasonable night, I was now worried about any my right foot, as it was quite swollen, in fact it had ballooned. The staff explained that as I was on a drip there was a lot of fluid in my system, which had caused the foot to swell.

However, I was able to get up and have a shower and then I went for yet another chest X-ray. At this stage I was managing to get out of the bed and into a wheelchair during the day.

My brother arrived from New Zealand on Wednesday, 14 May, on his first of three visits. He fussed over me; buying me food that I felt like from the cafeteria, such as boiled eggs.

Unfortunately, the whole time he was there I was mainly asleep, or dozing on and off all day, and when he did bring my eggs I couldn't eat them. I felt so embarrassed but he realized I was not well, and during that time there were only a few days that he saw me fully awake.

On Tuesday, 20 May I had a meeting with St Margaret's Rehabilitation Hospital personnel to finalize the details regarding my move to the rehabilitation hospital. I was advised on Wednesday, 21 May that I would be moving by ambulance, the following morning between10 and 11am and on Thursday, 22 May I was transferred by ambulance from the Queen Elizabeth Hospital to the St Margaret Hospital in Adelaide.

Summary of Electronic Tests:

22 April 2014: Attached to Heart monitor

23 April 2014: X-ray left foot

23 April 2014: CT Left foot

1 May 2014: Chest X-ray

7 May 2014: Ultra sound left shoulder

12 May 2014: Bladder scan

13 May 2014: Chest X-ray

13 May 2014: Ultra sound right leg

20 May 2014: Chest X-ray

25 July 2014: Chest X-ray

7 August 2014: Ultra sound left Shoulder

3 October 2014: Chest X-ray

9 October 2014: CT of Body

30 January 2015: CT of Body

26 August 2015: Ultra sound abdomen

12 December 2015: X-ray left Knee

Summary of Operations:

24 April 2014: Bone Marrow

25 April 2014: Top of left leg to unblock artery

26 April 2014: Left leg calf muscle to unblock artery

27 April 2014: Left Leg Amputate foot

5 May 2014: Picc Line Operation #1

10 July 2014: Picc Line Operation #2

14 July 2014: Picc Line Operation #3

7 August 2014: Picc Line Operation #4

9 October 2014: Bone Marrow

Summary of Blood Transfusions:

5 June 2014: Blood 1x Unit

11 June 2014: Blood 1x Unit

23 July 2014: Blood 1x Unit

24 July 2014: Blood 1x Unit

25 July 2014: Blood 2x Unit

15 Sept 2014: Blood 1x Unit

16 Sept 2014: Blood 2x Unit

Chapter 7

Saint Margaret Hospital

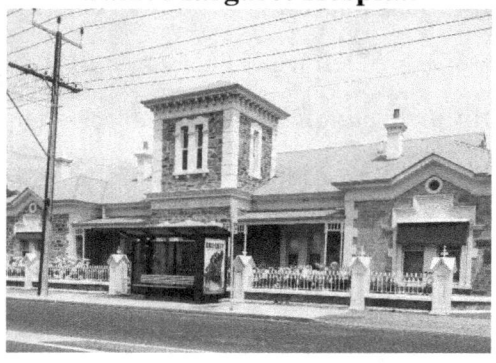

Saint Margaret Hospital is a small Rehabilitation Hospital in Adelaide, South Australia

Thursday, 22 May I have been transferred by Ambulance from the Queen Elizabeth Hospital to the St Margaret Hospital in Adelaide

Similar Ambulance that transported me from Queen Elizabeth hospital to St Margaret Hospital.

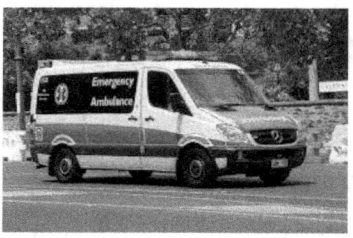

On 22 May 2014 I arrived at the St Margaret hospital by ambulance, from the Queen Elizabeth Hospital, and was taken to my own private room.

It felt as if I was being fussed over due to my having Chemotherapy treatment for my Lymphoma, although I was actually there for rehabilitation for my amputation.

My room was quite large, being self-contained with a shower and toilet, and with French doors, and windows overlooking the front of the hospital.

The hospital supplied me with a special water bed which stirred the water over and over, like a continuously moving mattress massaging me in order to prevent bedsores developing. Unfortunately, it also had a noisy pump!

I was supplied with this mattress, as Chemotherapy treatment patients tend to lay in bed, sleeping and resting, day after day. If I had only been admitted for rehabilitation I would not have been provided with the special mattress, as I would normally have been up and about every day.

The standard rehabilitation period for amputation is six weeks, plus or minus, depending on the individual's progress. Due to my Chemotherapy treatment, I had to be isolated from the other patients, as the Chemotherapy treatment affects and weakens the immune system, making me extremely vulnerable to infections/diseases. My meals were taken in my room for the same reason.

As I was going to be there for a few weeks I wanted to be comfortable, and I had my son buy me a small stereo with a remote. My son also installed my TV, which had a CD player for playing DVD movies.

I was also assigned my own wheelchair so that I could wheel myself around the hospital and outside, but had to be careful not to get any infections. Most of the time I wore a mask, and the nurses also wore masks when around me to lessen the risk of infection.

At this stage I was feeling quite well, except for some days when due to the Chemotherapy, I would wake up very tired and stay in bed all day. Other days I would feel fine and hop into my wheelchair, scooting around the corridors of the hospital. If the sun was shining, and it was not too cold I would also venture outside.

Each morning the nurse would come in with clean towels for my shower and offer to shower me, but I always managed to shower myself (well 95% of the time); not because I was embarrassed, but because I felt I wanted to be independent.

The breakfast would be delivered to my room, after my shower, which meant that I was spoilt, and I was given the opportunity to order boiled or poached eggs, which was a privilege. This was due to the fact I had lost a lot of weight, and was down to 55 kg whereas I was normally over 80 kg.

They needed to build me up, to increase my stamina, and ward off any chance of infection of any description, whilst I was undergoing Chemotherapy.

Each day, with breakfast, the nurse gave me my medication, consisting of several pills. The nurses would also dress my stump wound every day, until I took over and was able to dress it myself, which saved them time and also gave me something to do.

I listened to the radio all day and sometimes at night as well, as I was a little lonely. My family and friends would visit me at night and during the weekend, but the days were long. I also had my iPhone and iPad with me and I spent a lot of time on the Internet and Facebook. I bought DVDs on eBay and had them sent to the hospital, playing them on my TV, which had an internal DVD player.

David, my Physiotherapist, would visit around 10am each day, and if I was feeling fine and not too tired, he would have me doing exercises in my room. As time went on and I became stronger, I was able to do my exercises in the hospital gymnasium.

Up until this point I had not been eating very well at all, but on Sunday, 25 May, they served me a roast lamb lunch, with mint sauce, roast potatoes, pumpkin and cauliflower. I remember eating it all, so my appetite had returned.

At this stage, my son and I decided that it would not be possible for me return to Brinkworth to live in my caravan, in the near future. My son sold both the caravan and my Navara Ute, which I used for towing the caravan.

He then found a flat near the Queen Elizabeth Hospital, but first we had to see if the flat was suitable for me and my wheelchair. The Director of Physiotherapy, Melisa, needed to accompany me to the flat to assess its suitability, and that I would be able to manage by myself. We arranged to view it in about a weeks' time.

On 30th May, 2014, the Oncology Nurse, Vinnie arrived at Saint Margaret Hospital from the Queen Elizabeth Hospital to start my second round of Chemotherapy treatment. She attached a bottle of Chemotherapy to me, and connected a small tube to the PICC line in my arm. She also gave me Chemotherapy pills to take for four days, and a day later gave me an injection into the stomach, which seemed to set the whole Chemotherapy process into action.

For the first few days after the Chemotherapy, in fact for the first week, I was very lethargic, and felt nauseated*, which meant I would miss my Physiotherapy exercises and sleep all day. *(This is detailed in length in the Chemotherapy Treatment Chapter)

As time went on I managed to complete all the exercises asked of me, and sometimes more than was required. I was beginning to regain my strength and self-confidence, as well as gaining weight. Not a lot of weight, but enough, however, I was still a very long way from getting a prosthetic leg.

At this stage I was finding my way around the hospital, and I discovered that they had their own laundry with washing machines and dryers, which the patients could use. I would get up early and beat everybody to the room, doing my washing and using the dryer once or twice a week. This was something more to do, and kept me active and independent. This also meant that I didn't have to give my dirty washing to my family.

During my explorations, I also found two vending machines in the patient dining room, at the other end of the hospital. One had food snacks, and the other was a coffee machine. This was great as I liked my coffee.

My son had organized a drawer full of coins for me which meant I could get up, even in the middle of the night, and wheel myself down (in the semi darkness) to the coffee vending machine

The biggest problem was wheeling myself back in my wheelchair with a mug full of hot coffee, (which I had to hold it between my legs), as I needed both hands to wheel myself. As well as the coffee, I often bought food snacks from the vending machine, although there was not a great selection, but it was good when you had no other option.

The role of the Director of Physiotherapy was to teach me how I could live independently and manage safely at home.

Melisa and David taught me how to get onto the bed, the toilet, and how to get into the shower, and shower myself. These may sound simple activities, but it's not that easy;

the trick is to how you perform a swiveling action, and then sit down.

The only time I was ever embarrassed whilst in any of the five hospitals, and having been showered by many nurses, was when I was asked by Melisa, the Director of Physiotherapy, to shower myself in front of her. She needed to be satisfied that I could manage on my own at home. I understood why, and this was not a problem; but as she was in corporate dress as a Director, and not in uniform I felt more self-conscious. I was not uncomfortable about it, just not sure how I felt. As well as all of the above, I also had to prove to my Physiotherapist that I could manage on one leg, and use my wheelchair. I was given some tests to demonstrate my ability.

Firstly, I had to stand on one leg for as long as I could, and I surprised the Physiotherapist, and myself, by standing for 15 minutes. Next was a test where I had to follow the Physiotherapist, in my wheelchair, along the street footpath for two blocks, crossing back and forth as we went. We then turned and went a further two blocks, also crossing several times and then turned, proceeding a further two blocks whilst crossing several times, until we had done the full circuit of four blocks and back to the hospital. This was very tiring but I was determined to succeed, as I knew if I failed the tests, that they would not discharge me.

After having demonstrated I could shower, dry and dress myself; wheel myself around in my wheelchair, cross streets; move from my wheelchair on one leg to a chair; wash and dry my clothes in the hospital laundry, Melisa, the Director of Physiotherapy advised I had passed all the tests, and gave me the okay to be able to look after myself.

On 2nd June, 2014 I was advised that I could look at the flat that my son had found for me, to see if it was suitable. Melisa arranged for me to go by a disability Access Taxi to the flat the following day.

After four days, my Chemotherapy bottle was empty on June 3rd, and was removed by my Chemotherapy nurse, who came from the Queen Elizabeth Hospital. She also gave me pills, plus an injection in my stomach which I understood set off the Chemotherapy process.

Later that day, along with my Director of Physiotherapy, I travelled by Access Taxi in my wheelchair and viewed the flat, checking how I would be able to manage.

Firstly, the kitchen to see how I would manage cupboards, the cooking and dishes, etc. Then the dining room; followed by the laundry, toilet, bathroom and finally, the bedroom. I was able to access all in my wheelchair, and managed all the areas with no problems.

My Director of Physiotherapy was happy, and signed off on the flat's suitability, providing that I fitted a couple of extra hand rails in the toilet and shower, plus a ramp for my wheelchair at the front door. Then my son confirmed with the landlord that I wanted to lease the flat, with the date to be confirmed when the hospital had settled on a discharge date.

I awoke on the 5th June, feeling really flat, even too tired to shower (and I love my shower), so I lay in bed all day.

After considering my condition the hospital decided to give me a blood transfusion that afternoon, plus a second the next day. As they began giving me the blood transfusion my temperature spiked, and they stopped, as a precaution. Later they resumed the blood transfusion, which takes a total of four hours, and all went well.

The following day the nurse arrived from Queen Elizabeth hospital and administered my second blood transfusion without a hitch. I was now feeling much better, after the two blood transfusions.

I then enquired if I would be able to be to get out of the hospital for a period of time over the weekend. I had begun to plan my future, and I had decided that I needed to buy a new small two door car as most two door cars have large doors providing space to store a wheel chair behind the driver's seat. This meant that I would be able to put the wheelchair in and out of the car.

Searching online I found a car to look at, which was some distance from the hospital. I arranged to get a pass for a few hours out of the hospital and my son came to take me to see this car. It happened to be raining that day just to make it more difficult, as I was in the wheelchair. As it turned out the car wasn't suitable, so back to the motel (hospital) we went.

Once again, I awoke on 9th June, with little stamina. I only ate a little bit of bread with some olive oil, as I was very tired, and not feeling the best.

My Specialist Rehabilitation Physician came to visit on 10 June, and advised that the following week, I would be going for the first cast of my stump, to make a prosthetic leg. Usually the prosthetic would have been made, and I'd learn to use it and walk whilst in the rehabilitation hospital. However, due to my Chemotherapy treatment having many side effects, primarily hindering the healing process of my stump, the fitting of my prosthetic leg was being hindered.

By 11th June I must have felt better, but hungry as I asked my son if he could pick me up some Kentucky fried chicken and chips, and a frozen Coke, which went down a treat. However, the following day I was once again very flat and tired; another day to just stay in bed.

My Specialist Rehabilitation Physician again visited on 13th June, for his normal checks, and confirmed I could go out of the Hospital on the weekend for four hours, for some welcome recreation.

My son picked me up at 10am on the 14th and wheeled me around the shopping centre in my wheelchair. However, I felt helpless and wished I could have done more. Returning to the hospital I was really tired and went to sleep almost immediately.

On Sunday, 15th June, I was feeling depressed and felt I needed a breakthrough in my life. I made my mind up that I would get out of hospital and into my flat as soon as possible, as I felt I could get more exercise and generally feel better.

Although I did not have my prosthetic leg by Monday, 16th June my Physiotherapist, David, fitted a temporary prosthesis and, with the aid of a walking frame, I walked for the first time on two legs. It was a good feeling, but was short lived as unknown to me at time I was to be in my wheelchair until November, due to all the problems associated with the Chemotherapy.

Later that day I asked the hospital doctor and the Director of Physiotherapy if I could be discharged on Friday, 20th June. I was advised that I needed to ask my Specialist doctor who was coming the next day.

Well, overnight at 3am, on 17th June, I had my first fall whilst sitting on side of the bed, reaching out in the dark for my wee bottle. I slipped and fortunately my shoulder hit the bedside cabinet, saving me from falling hard. I ended up on the floor and luckily, I was unhurt; oh well then, this one-legged man had to get back in bed! What, call nurse? No, I didn't want them to know at this late stage.

That morning the Specialist arrived from the Queen Elizabeth Hospital and I asked if it was possible for me to be discharged on Friday. He advised that he was having a meeting whilst at the hospital, and would let me know. Later that morning I was advised that they had agreed to discharge me on Friday.

This was great news, as the normal rehabilitation term is six weeks and I was being discharged in just four weeks. However, I had at this stage been in a hospital (one of five) for a total of eleven weeks, and did not know that stage I was yet to be admitted to the Queen Elizabeth hospital twice more for a week, due to my Chemotherapy knocking me around.

They advised they were sending me for a stump fitting for my prosthetic leg on Wednesday, plus an appointment on Friday for my third round of Chemotherapy at the Queen Elizabeth Hospital at 11:30am.

I leased the flat from the Thursday so that my belongings could be moved from storage, and so that the fridge and kitchen could be stocked before I move there on the Friday, after my Chemotherapy. I also needed an access ramp to be built over the front deck for it to be level with the front door.

On Wednesday, 18th June. I went by Access Taxi to Prostek, the prosthetic suppliers, where my Prosthetist, Bridie, took a plaster cast of my stump and measured my other leg, to match the prosthetic.

My things were moved from storage into my flat on Thursday, 19th June, and the fridge and freezer were stocked with food and beer.

I was discharged from St Margaret's hospital at 11am on Friday, 20th June and transported by Access Taxi for the short trip to the Queen Elizabeth Hospital for the commencement of my third round of Chemotherapy and then home to my flat.

Discharged from Saint Margaret's Hospital Friday, 20 June 2014

Chapter Eight

Home in My Flat

After three months, on the 20th June 2014, I finally made it out of Hospital and home to my new flat.

It has a Lounge, Kitchen, Dining room, two Bedrooms, Bathroom, and a Garage, which are all very roomy making it suitable for my wheelchair.

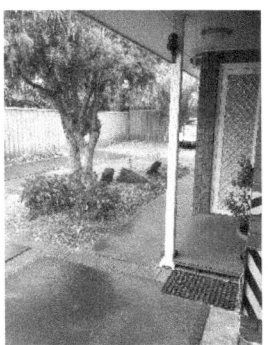 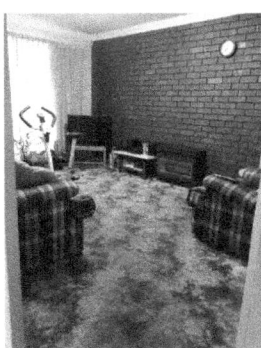

Front Door   ***Lounge***

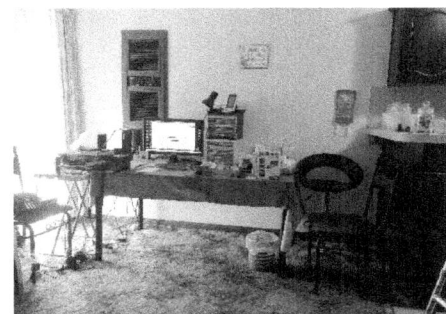 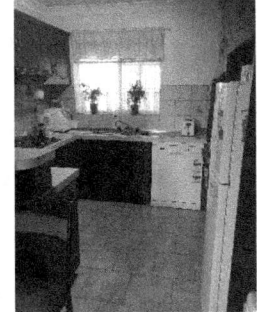

Dining Room   *Kitchen*

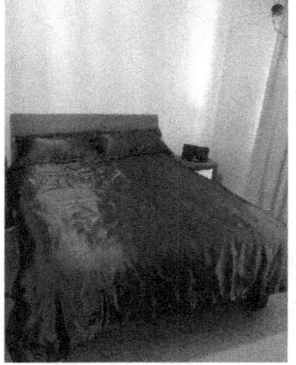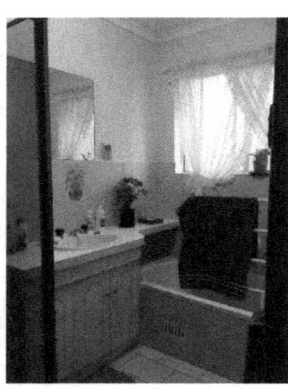

Master Bedroom   *Bathroom*

On Friday 20 June 2014, I wheeled myself across the road from the Queen Elizabeth Hospital and arrived home at my new flat; after the commencement of my third round of Chemotherapy medication and with the Chemotherapy bottle connected.

My son had made and fitted a plywood deck to raise the front veranda floor level to the height of the entrance door.

Then he needed to build a ramp from the driveway to the deck and I helped where I could, by holding this and that, and a week or so later I painted it myself. With the ramp and deck completed I had complete wheelchair access, to and from the flat.

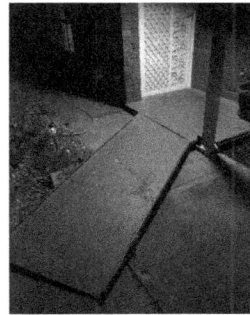
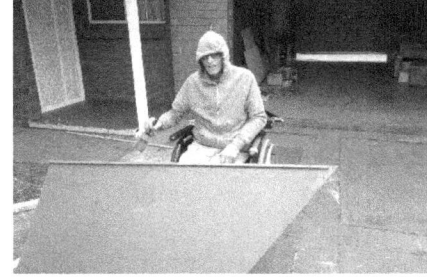

Wheelchair Ramp   ***Myself Painting the Ramp***

When I had finished painting the ramp, I sat down and relaxed with a beer, feeling very relieved as even though I was in a wheelchair, I once gain had my freedom and independence. Although I was in a wheelchair I could do the things I wanted to do, plus I could go out where and when I wanted.

My next challenge was to buy myself a small car suitable for my situation, plus accommodate a wheelchair behind the front seat. It was convenient that it was my left leg which was amputated, as this allowed me to drive an automatic car without any modifications.

By Saturday the 21st June I was relaxed, and looked on the Internet for cars for sale, finding three cars that I was interested in having a look at. As there was a taxi stand directly outside my home I hired a taxi and went looking at cars, in my wheelchair. I found a small Alfa Romeo two door, and the car salesperson was kind enough to test putting my wheelchair in the car while I sat in a chair. It looked like the car I wanted except that particular one had a problem with the paintwork, which would cost a lot of money to repair.

I cooked myself a nice meal, on Sunday 22nd June, a T-Bone steak and veggies, as I was starting to feel fatigued and tired. It was a great feeling to be able to do things for myself again, especially cooking.

On leaving the Hospital the Dietitian had given me an 'eat anything' diet, including heaps of butter and fats to aid me putting on weight, as I was only 55kg at this stage and normally I weighed 80kg. They considered it more important for me to put on weight, than worry about my cholesterol level, as I needed the stamina and energy during my Chemotherapy treatment.

Over the weekend, I looked for cars for sale on the internet and found an Alfa Romeo, the same model as the cars on private sale. I contacted them and they were kind enough to offer to bring the car to me to look at, so I arranged to see the car on the Monday. The car was brought to me to inspect, and after taking it for a test drive, I purchased it there and then with the cash my son had withdrawn from my bank account for me. I then rang and insured it immediately.

The car was ideal as it was small enough for me to drive around the city and handle generally, as well as fitting in the garage perfectly with room enough to enable me to get in and out of the car, and into my wheelchair. Being a two-door model it has large doors so I could push my driver seat forward, fold up the wheelchair, slide it in behind the seat to store, then bring the seat forward again, as in photos below.

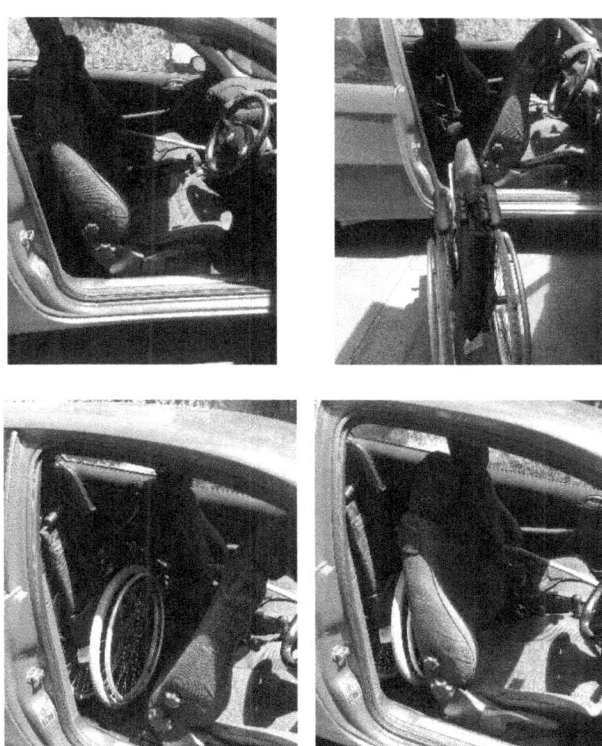

Wheelchair fitting snug in behind the front seat

Unfortunately, I could not always drive due to the effects of the Chemotherapy treatment, so I always waited until late in the Chemotherapy cycle, and as long as I felt okay and 'with it' I would go for a drive.

A woman from Domiciliary Care (a Government department for domestic care.) came to visit me on Tuesday, 24th June, to check if I was comfortable with everything, after moving in to my flat.

She had organised a hand rail to be fitted in the toilet plus one in the shower and had organised a loan wheelchair, a walking frame, and a toilet raise (raises toilet seat to a level equal to the wheel chair). I now had two wheelchairs; one on loan, and the other my own, which allowed me to have one permanently in the car.

She also arranged regular cleaning of my flat including cleaning the kitchen, the benchtops, mopping all the tiled floors, vacuuming carpets, cleaning the toilet and shower, making the bed and doing the washing.

Being winter and quite cold, which was exacerbated by the effects of the Chemotherapy treatment, I was wearing a jersey plus a jacket. While I was talking to her I was feeling hot so I decided to take off my jacket, and as my Chemotherapy bottle tube was threaded through my sleeve I unintentionally pulled out the Chemotherapy line leading down to my heart.

The Chemotherapy solution spilled, and this was a problem. I folded the pipe straight away so the Chemotherapy couldn't run out anymore and immediately rang the hospital. They sent the Oncology home service nurse Vinnie, who happened to be at the Queen Elizabeth Hospital, straight across the road from my flat. She came over and cleaned up the Chemotherapy that had been spilt (By using the emergency materials, gloves and a gown stored in my flat) and made it all safe, plus removed the bottle of Chemotherapy.

She then arranged for me to go back over to the hospital so they could complete my Chemotherapy plus organise an appointment for the surgeons to operate and fit a new PICC (Percutaneous Indwelling Central Catheter) line.

At this stage the stump had still not fully healed, due to the Chemotherapy which affects the immune system, and the body's healing properties. The RDNS (Royal District Nursing Service) home service, came to my home twice a week for several weeks and dressed the wound until the stump finally healed. They also left a Kit of cleaning aids and dressings; so that everything was on hand each time they came and enabled me to dress it myself on the other days.

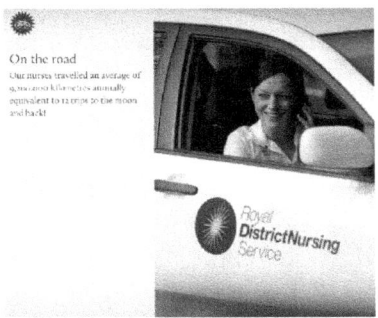

RDNS Service

I wanted to set the flat up to suit my personal requirements. Firstly, I needed to automate my garage roller door so I could open it with a remote. I purchased a unit from my local hardware and my son and I installed it, which made things much easier for me, as I was still in the wheelchair and at that stage did not have my prosthetic leg.

I had a small 3mx3m shed on my block at Brinkworth and I had some friends who disassembled it for me and brought it to my flat and reassembled it with also help from my son. I installed some benches in the shed and hung all my tools on the wall, and fitted a light. Then I built myself another ramp for the back door, so that I could get in and out through the back door to the shed in my wheelchair.

I also set up my computer, which is my main hobby, in my dining room. Being in a wheelchair, it was difficult to stand at the sink on one leg and wash the dishes, so I installed a dish washer to make life easier. Some days I would wake up and just feel tired and very flat, so I would just stay in bed all day; sometimes even for several days.

At this stage I really needed help, and my son and daughter-in-law were both working, plus they had already put so much energy into looking after me I felt they needed a break. I asked one of my brothers to help out, and early in August he came over from New Zealand for a second time. He looked after me for about ten days; cooking meals and taking me out in my car, driving me around, and wheeling me around in my wheel chair, including going to the QEH for appointments.

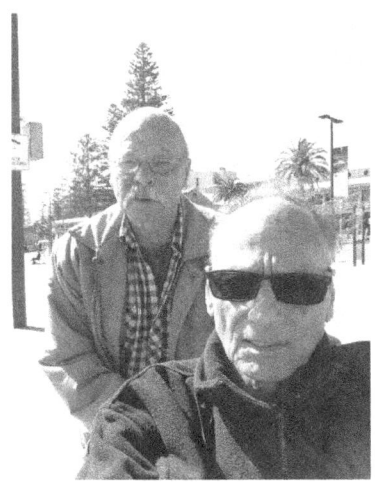

Photo of my Brother pushing me around in wheelchair

September the third was my 75th birthday and my son organized to have dinner at the local hotel. As a surprise, he invited people I had not seen for a while including workmates, and Donna, my daughter came from New Zealand for a third visit to look after me, as well as my grandson Ryan (Donna's son) came from Sydney.

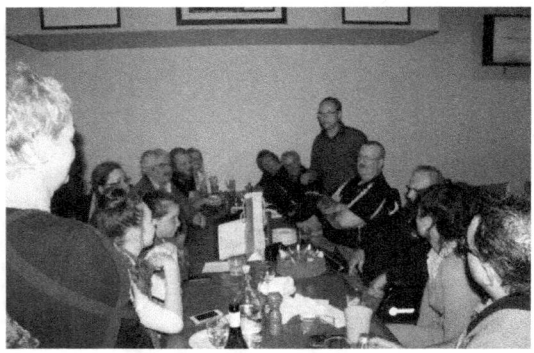

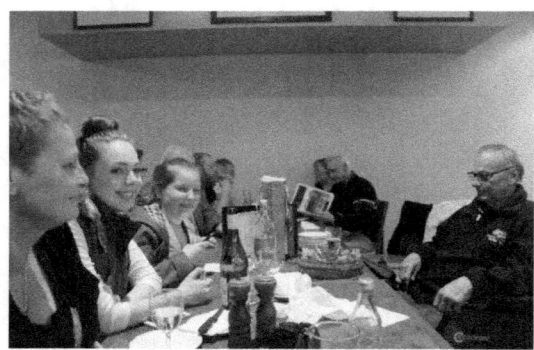

Photos of my 75th Birthday at the local Hotel

Once again, I was looked after impeccably.

One day my daughter drove us in my car to Kangaroo Island (an Island two hours from Adelaide). We crossed to the island on the one hour ferry trip then drove around sightseeing before returning on the ferry and driving home to my flat.

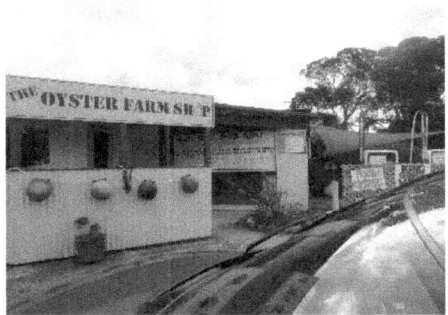

Oyster Shop on Kangaroo Island

The highlight of the trip was finding a fishery on the coast, and gorging ourselves on nice fresh oysters, plus taking some home for later.

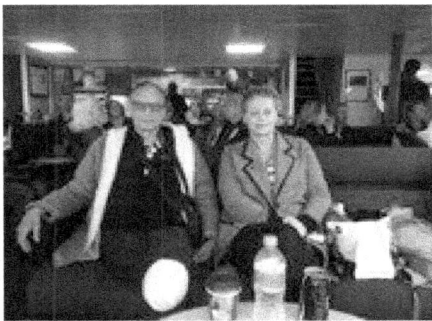

My Daughter and I on the Ferry

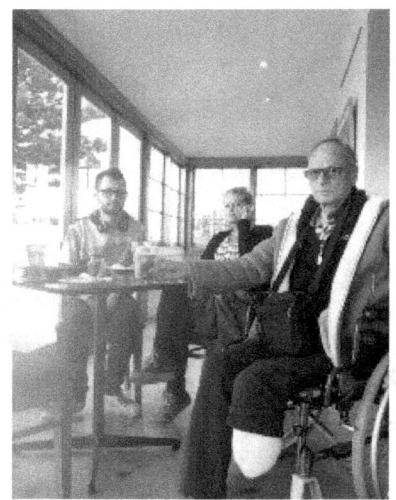

Ryan, Donna and myself

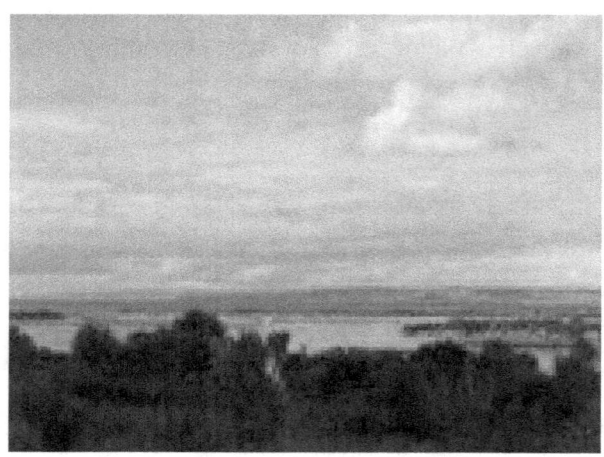

A view of Kangaroo Island

I still needed help for most of my daily living including getting groceries plus preparing meals. My wife Gail, from whom I was separated, was kind enough to sometimes come twice a week to help by driving from the country for two hours, and driving back to her home later in the day.

She brought me prepared meals and we would go to the supermarket and buy groceries, and drive to the beach to walk one of the dogs, the Boxer Blake or Case, whichever she bought with her. Both dogs have now passed on, having lived to great ages.

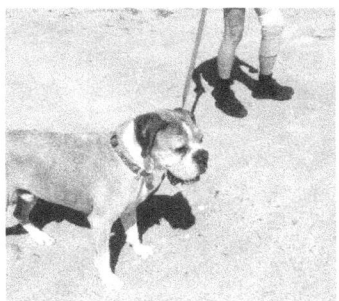

Case

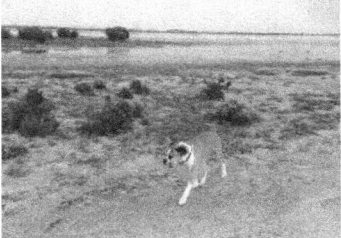

Blake

I then contacted my stepdaughter Lisa, who lives in New Zealand, and asked if she would be able to come and help me, so she travelled from New Zealand on 20th September, and looked after me for ten days. She completely cleaned my Flat plus cooked meals (fattening me up as I desperately needed to put on weight); taking me grocery shopping, and for outings to places such as a day at Glenelg beach as per the photos.

This was such a great help, although while she was there I spent many days sleeping, still experiencing the effects of the Chemotherapy treatment.

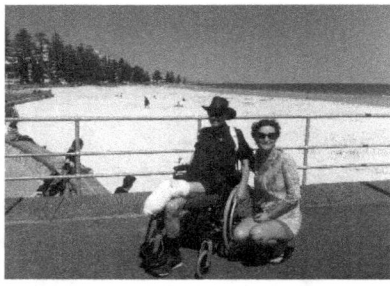

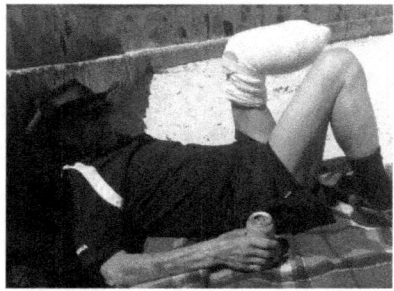

At Glenelg Beach Adelaide

Chapter Nine

My Chemotherapy Story

I was advised by my Haematologist of my Chemotherapy Treatment Program on Tuesday, 6th May 2014. This was to be comprised of six rounds of Chemotherapy treatment, with the dosage being increased by twenty per cent from and including round four, (sounds like a boxing match and it turned out to be very similar). Each round was to be over three weeks, a total period of eighteen weeks, which became nineteen weeks.

At this stage I was in the Queen Elizabeth Hospital Cancer ward and I was taken by wheelchair to the floor above, to the Cancer Clinic, where the Chemotherapy Treatment is administered. The Hospital Pharmacist then came and went over all my medication explaining what each pill/tablet did, the dosage and frequency.

Note: all Chemotherapy treatment items and pills plus all the equipment and items such as gloves and plastic gowns are colored Purple/Violet.

Prior to this I had had an operation where they installed a connection in the top of my arm called a Percutaneous Indwelling Central Catheter (PICC line).

I was given a local anesthetic for the operation, where a small hose was inserted into my arm up through my shoulder and down to my heart, using Ultrasound to guide them to place it correctly. It was completed by fitting a snap connection to the end of the hose to allow for future Chemotherapy/ Blood/ Intervenes procedures.

The seal around my connection to my arm required redressing every 7 days, in order to keep it clean after showers etc., and the Oncology nurse would replace the dressing on her regular visits.

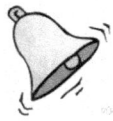 **DONG, Round 1**

Chemotherapy Treatment, 6th May 2014
On the 6th May I was prepped for my first round of Chemotherapy treatment which became, well what would you say, a reality or a nightmare?

The Cancer Clinic was abuzz with professionalism, humor and just plain lovely staff. The atmosphere was relaxing and nonchalant regarding what was about to happen. I was waited on with drinks, nice food and pleasantness all round.

There were many very large comfortable chairs to sit for preparation, and administering the Chemotherapy medication, as in the following photo.

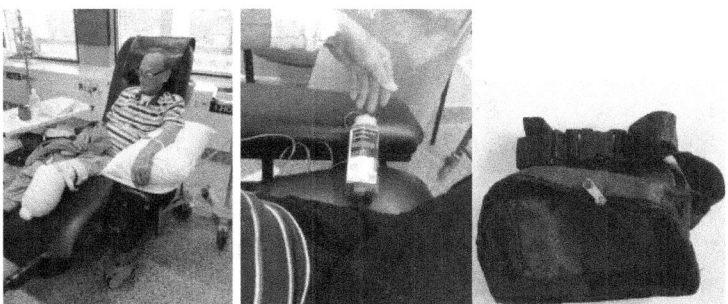

Above I am sitting in the large chair with the Chemotherapy bottle attached with the small hose leading to the connection in my arm plus the bag used to hold the Chemotherapy bottle for the four days of each round of treatment

Firstly, the staff explained the procedure, and then gave me something, (not sure what), after which I had to wait for some time like an hour.

Then the Chemotherapy bottle was connected to my PICC line, and I was given a small waist bag (To hold the Chemotherapy bottle). They then put the small Chemotherapy bottle into the bag, which had a small hose from it connecting to the PICC Line in my arm. It was explained I would wear this for four days, being the period for the Chemotherapy to automatically inject into my blood flow.   At this stage I also had to take several Chemotherapy pills twice a day, for four days as per my medication schedule.

All was fine until my left arm became swollen, and they stopped the Chemotherapy injection. I am not sure why, however they restarted the Chemotherapy the following day on the 7th May, 2016 and all was well. After a total of four days (I was still in the Cancer ward of QEH) they removed the empty Chemotherapy bottle and administered an injection into my stomach prompting the Chemotherapy reaction.

During the following days leading up to my second round of Chemotherapy I was feeling quite well, and I was thinking, as one does, that this is a piece of cake! Mm, how wrong can one be?

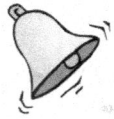 **DONG, Round 2**

Chemotherapy Treatment 30th May 2014
On 30th May, 2014 the Home services Oncology Nurse, Vinnie, arrived at Saint Margaret Hospital from the Queen Elizabeth Hospital to start my second round of Chemotherapy treatment by attaching a bottle of Chemotherapy to me and connecting a small tube to my PICC line in my arm. She also giving me Chemotherapy pills as per my medication schedule to take for the following four days.

The Oncology Nurse returned on 3rd June, and removed my empty Chemotherapy bottle, giving me an injection in the stomach which set the whole Chemotherapy process into action. She also replaced the PICC line dressing. Over the following two weeks the seal was replaced by the nurses at the Saint Margaret Hospital.

After the Chemotherapy, the first few days were fine, and then I would start to feel very lethargic, tired and nauseated.

From this time on I would have good days and bad days, mainly extremely tired, so I would miss the physio exercises and sleep all day.

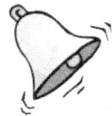 **DONG, Round 3**

Chemotherapy Treatment 20th June 2014

On 20th June, I was discharged from the Saint Margaret Hospital and an Access cab took me back to the Queen Elizabeth Hospital (QEH) for my third round of Chemotherapy treatment. I was prepped in the large comfortable chairs, whilst they connected the Chemotherapy bottle to my PICC line, and then the bottle went into the bag for the next four days, along with my medication as per the schedule.

Later that day I moved into my flat across the road from the QEH. It was great to be out of hospital, and I was starting to get the hang of things with the Chemotherapy procedure. Then on the 24th June a woman from Domiciliary Care visited, and being winter and cold, I had a jersey plus a jacket on. (Remember that I was also on Chemotherapy treatment at this time) Whilst I was talking to her I was feeling hot, so I decided to take off my jacket and as my Chemotherapy bottle tube was threaded through my sleeve, I unintentionally pulled out the Chemotherapy line leading down to my heart.

The Chemotherapy spilled, and this was a problem. I folded the pipe straight away so the Chemotherapy couldn't run out anymore, and I immediately contacted the Queen Elizabeth Hospital. My Oncology Home Service Nurse, Vinnie, came over and cleaned up the Chemotherapy that had been spilt (Using emergency materials, gloves and a gown stored in my flat) making it all safe, plus removing the bottle of Chemotherapy.

She then arranged for me to go back over to the hospital so they could complete my Chemotherapy, and organise an appointment for the surgeons to operate and fit a new PICC line. The effects of the Chemotherapy by this time had well and truly set in, and over the following two weeks I spent many days in bed. I was lucky enough to have people caring for me in one way or another.

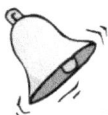

DONG, Round 4

Chemotherapy Treatment 11th July 2014

Well this round, the Chemotherapy dosage was increased by twenty per cent, as previously planned.

I went to the Queen Elizabeth Hospital Cancer Clinic, and I was prepped for my fourth round of Chemotherapy treatment, as per the previous visits. I then wheeled myself home and all was fine. I was having a good weekend until around 8am on Sunday the 13th July, when I was having a shower. Somehow the PICC line came adrift, and the small hose leading to the heart pulled part way out!

So, I did a temporary fix, got dressed and then, yes wheeled myself over to the Queen Elizabeth Hospital Emergency Department. It was only 9am, and a Sunday so luckily, they were not busy. The staff on that morning was not experienced with Chemotherapy so they called for someone from the Cancer ward to assist. The nurse that came was one that had attended me when I was in the Cancer ward so she knew what to do, which was unfortunately to remove the Chemotherapy line completely. This now meant I had to have another operation to fit a new PICC line. (The third time)

Due to the Chemotherapy, only being connected for a day they made an urgent appointment for the next day to have a new PICC line fitted.

On the Monday, I had the operation fitting the new PICC line, which allowed me to complete the Chemotherapy round and then on the 18th July the Oncology Nurse, Vinnie, came and gave me my injection.

Now remember the strength of the Chemotherapy had been increased by twenty per cent, and within two hours of having the injection to set off the process I was flat out in bed. I felt terrible, really, really, terrible. It felt like every muscle in my body was aching, and like a bad bout of flu'. My son contacted the hospital but there was nothing they could do, I just had to ride it out.

The treatment was now starting to take its toll and I became very emotional every day, and remained that way until early in 2015. I was advised that it was a characteristic of the treatment. I had many appointments with my Clinical Psychologist, Sarah, whom helped me through the difficult times. (More in details in the Appendices).

On the 24th July, just six days after the injection, my mouth became full of sores to the point I could not talk or eat. I was truly a mess. My son contacted the hospital and he took me to the Cancer Clinic. Once there the nurses called a doctor and he immediately admitted me to the Cancer Ward. (My twelfth week of hospitalisation)

Back in Queen Elizabeth Hospital Cancer Ward

The following days were hell as I was in a lot of pain. The doctors administered pain killers but nothing seemed to help until they tried a pain killer called Endone; yes, it finally worked and I had pain relief. However, it was short lived as it only worked for an hour or two, but I was saved, as they said I could have it regularly. The biggest problem with Chemotherapy is that you lose your healing capacity, so it was nearly a week before my mouth healed sufficiently for me to go home. Then a side effect of the Endone was constipation, which in turn blocked my urine flow, so then I had to have a Catheter fitted to relieve that problem.

I was discharged at midday on the 29th July, and I wheeled myself home to my flat across the road from the QEH. The horrible side effects of the Chemotherapy were hanging on at this stage, so I spent more days in bed than out of bed, where the effects of the past rounds had by this time had diminished.

Then, you would not believe it, yes, I was having a shower and yet again the PICC line came adrift; so back to the QEH for my fourth PICC line operation. Very embarrassing and very demoralising.

As I am writing this I just ask myself how did I ever cope and get through all this; and I am a long way from finishing this story, and it's hard not to shed a tear whilst remembering these difficult times.

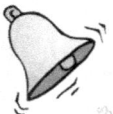

DONG, Round 5

Chemotherapy Treatment 8ᵗʰ August 2014

It is fair to say that I was not yet over the fourth round of Chemotherapy, when here I was lined up for another round at the Queen Elizabeth Hospital, Cancer Clinic.

I was prepped for my fifth round of treatment in the large comfortable chairs where you sit while they connect the Chemotherapy bottle to my PICC line, and then the bottle went into the bag for the next four days along with my Medication as per schedule. Then I would race home to my flat in my wheelchair, remember at this stage I did not yet have my Prosthetic leg.

The horrible effects of the treatment persisted with this round, and I spent days in bed feeling lifeless. Ten days later I needed to have several blood transfusions. Being so sick made me very depressed and I told my son that I refused to have round six of Chemotherapy. He made an appointment with the Oncology Doctor for me, and I explained how I felt. As a result, he suggested we delay the next round by two weeks. Having had the blood transfusion, I was feeling a little better so I made a deal to delay it one week to sort of "let's get it over with", (as I was thinking if I leave for two weeks I may never go back), so the new date for round six was 7th September

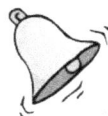

DONG, Round 6

Chemotherapy Treatment 7th Sept 2014

I was lined up for yet another round of Chemotherapy at the Queen Elizabeth Hospital, Cancer Clinic. I was prepped for my sixth round of Chemotherapy treatment with the same routine as previously, before returning to my flat.

Then, on 10th September, the Oncology Nurse, Vinnie, came to my flat as normal and gave me my injection. From then it was much the same, with the effects of the Chemotherapy sending me to bed for days on end; but as time passed I began to feel better.

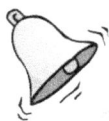

DONG, DONG, DONG

Chemotherapy Rounds Finished!!

Then on 3rd October, three weeks on from the finish of my Chemotherapy treatment, all the Lymphoma symptoms returned. I was having huge sweats several times during the night, I was also vomiting and my temperature was spiking around 40deg C. So back to the Queen Elizabeth Hospital Emergency Department where they called for a doctor from Oncology to examine me, and he advised me I was yet again being admitted.

Back in Queen Elizabeth Hospital Cancer Ward
The 3rd October was now the start of my thirteenth week in hospital. I only coped during this period by living each day as it came, never looking ahead much, just persevering with each problem, one at a time.

There was a problem with finding a bed and I was put in the Cardio Ward, for two days then moved to the Cancer Ward. I was moved to a special room that was pressurized, so that the doors were always closed, unlike all the rooms I had been in previously. This was because they considered that I had an infection; and to eliminate any chance of further infections.

At this stage I felt fine, and all was good apart from when I was having a shower when I stood on one leg to dry myself. I overbalanced and fell; crashing into the shower chair which broke my fall. Luckily the nurse was in my room and came running to find my naked body lying on the floor. Thankfully I was fine, and she helped me up, taking it all in her stride.

Then on the 8th October, the Oncologist sent me to the Royal Adelaide Hospital for yet another PET scan to ensure that I was clear of lymphoma, and then I returned to the QEH.

On the 9th October, I had another bone marrow operation plus I had a CT scan to ensure that I was clear of lymphoma.

After all the above tests the results showed I was clear of Lymphoma, and on the 10th October I was discharged from hospital.

Summary of Chemotherapy Treatment

The Haematologist advised that every three months/six months he would arrange for me to have blood tests followed by an appointment to examine and report my progress. At these appointments, he would physically examine me plus show and explain the results of my blood tests.

In summing up he always stated: *There is no cure for non-Hodgkin's Lymphoma and that it is very aggressive. He also went on to say if the Lymphoma returns it will be difficult to treat as they had already administered the strongest dosage of Chemotherapy that could be safely administered.*

He explained that any further treatment would only be effective if it is stronger than the previous treatment, therefore questioning the viability due to the strength required and the safety level.

The advice was *"just go and live life normally"*

Chapter 10

My Prosthetic Story

This chapter covers my Prosthetic history as a result of the amputation of my left foot.

After having my left foot amputated at the Queen Elizabeth Hospital on 28th April, 2014 I was transferred to the HDU (High Dependency Unit). On 1st May, 2014 a plaster cast was made to fit over my stump (as pictured below). This was a rigid casting to protect my stump, which was still healing, until I was fitted with a prosthetic leg.

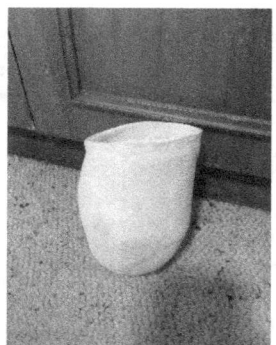 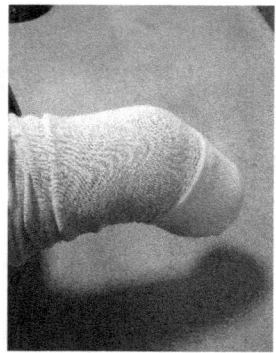

Plaster cast

A few weeks later on 18th June, 2014, whilst in Saint Margaret Hospital, I went by Access Cab for an appointment with my Prosthetist, Bridie, at "Prostek" a local company, (who specialize in Clinical Prosthetic and Orthotic Services) and had my first cast for a prosthetic leg.

I was discharged from the Saint Margaret Hospital on the 20th June, 2014 and on the 24th June I went back to Prostek for the first fitting of my prosthetic leg. The first cast was very basic, being just a socket attached to a pipe with a fixed rigid foot. This was a whole new experience, especially trying to adapt to the prosthetic leg, (pictured below).

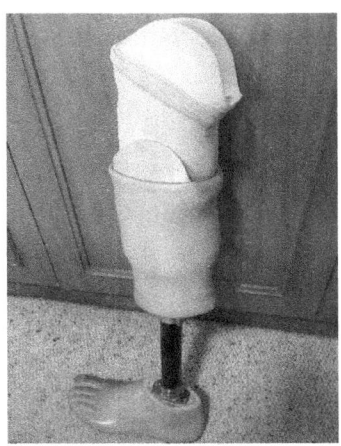

I was then assigned monthly appointments at the Queen Elizabeth Hospital with my Specialist Prosthetic Physician, and my Prosthetist, Bridie, for checkups and guidance. In addition, I was programmed for twice-weekly physiotherapy exercises for strengthening muscles and learning to walk with the leg.

I was not able to walk on the leg at this stage as I was having problems with the fitting as the swelling/wound of my wound had not healed, which was one of the side effects of still being on chemotherapy. It was decided, between myself and the Physiotherapy Department, that I would not use the leg until my chemotherapy treatment had finished, the last treatment being scheduled for the 7th September, 2014.

Having finished my Chemotherapy treatment on 1st October, 2014, my first prosthetic leg was finally refitted. I was now able to attend my twice-weekly physiotherapy at the Queen Elizabeth Hospital, in earnest. Fortunately, David, the Physiotherapist, was the same person whom had been my Physiotherapist at the St Margaret Hospital.

At each appointment, I would do exercises starting with the lying on a bed to build up my muscles in my arms and legs, then lifting hand weights for my arms, followed by lifting weights on a machine by pushing/stretching my legs. As the appointments continued on I was able to walk between a set of rails holding on to each rail at about hip height, then turning and doing exercises, similar to being on a see-saw. This was to teach and encourage balance. Next was walking with a frame; the frame being used as a safety device in case I lost my balance. Remember that these are very early stages for me in the rehabilitation process.

I bought myself an Exercycle and a walking frame so I could continue exercising at home as in photos below.

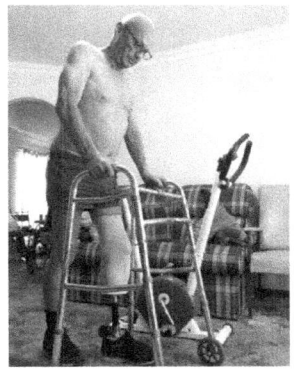
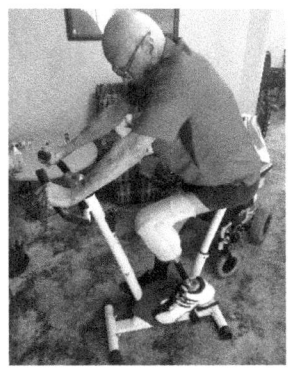

Walking with Frame   *Exercising Legs*

At this stage I was getting a sensation/hurting in my stump as I walked, but nothing was visible when removing the prosthetic. I found that my stump was very sensitive under the end, so I experimented and found by putting a gel cap, (made by cutting down a gel sock) over the end of the stump limited the discomfort.

This was a major step towards walking and I am still using the gel cap over the end of my stump. When using my 'wet leg' I use a single thickness gel cap, as in the photo.

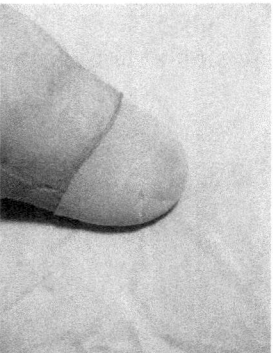

Cap used on Wet leg

For the next stage of physiotherapy, I used a walking stick to help me take the weight of my leg and steady myself; the more I walked the better I got.

My Physiotherapist advised me to massage the stump to help the circulation, and overall help the stump to settle, so I purchased a small hand held massage machine and massaged it every morning on the bed after my shower, and before getting dressed.

To me it seemed to help as I think it played a part in hardening the stump for the prosthetic leg.

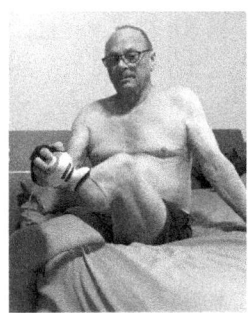
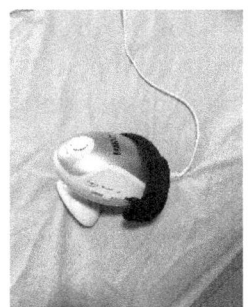

Massaging stump after shower   *The Massage device*

The next stage of physiotherapy required me to walk up a ramp to a platform, across the platform and down steps. Then I would turn and walk back up the steps, across the platform and down the ramp. On mastering this skill, the Physiotherapist took me outside to a grassed area, and had me walk on the grass. This was quite tricky as it was a little like walking on air, and hard to balance. On achieving the skills of learning to walk and balance, and doing the same at home, I was eventually assessed as good to go, as so my Physiotherapy appointments at the hospital were completed.

Time went on and as I gained strength my Prosthetic became uncomfortable, due to my stump being too tight in the socket.

I had planned, and booked, a trip to New Zealand in February 2015, but I was comfortable with the leg and still mainly in a wheelchair, so I cancelled the trip.

Then on 16th January, 2015 I went to Prostek, my prosthetic suppliers, and had a new cast made for a better fitting socket, with room for adjustment by way of using selected socks.

On 27th January, 2015 the prosthetic leg was fitted with the new socket, and I found it more comfortable and able to walk much easier..

At this time, I was still using my wheelchair for things such as showering, however my Specialist Doctor advised that I could have a new additional leg made for showering. So, on the 13th February, 2015 I went to Prostek and had another cast made, returning on the 12th March to have the leg fitted.

This 'wet leg' (I call it my shower leg), made life so much better and easier not having to wheel to the shower and sit in a chair to shower. Showering from a wheelchair is not easy as you have to crouch on one leg, swivel 180 degrees without slipping or falling, and sit in the shower chair. Then it is even more difficult to get out of the shower, (as you are now wet), by crouching and swiveling on one leg. I would have two towels; one on my wheelchair to sit on and the other on my bed, which I learnt to do in rehabilitation. The procedure was to sit on the towel in the wheelchair, roll into the bedroom to the bed, then once again crouch and swivel on one leg onto the bed, dry myself and then get dressed.

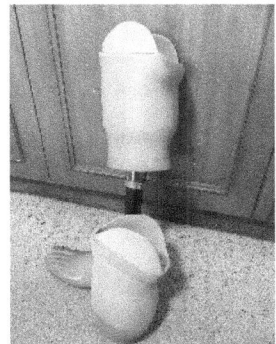 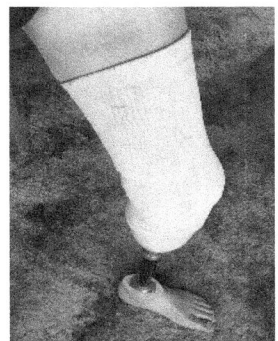

Wet Leg

I then made plans to travel to New Zealand for ten days, booking myself to travel in early May 2015. I took my shower leg but not my wheelchair, as most of the time I could manage without it.

The airline provided wheelchairs, and they transported me to and from the plane, and around the airports. All went well in New Zealand and I travelled comfortably.

My Specialist Prosthetic Physician advised they would be upgrading my prosthetic leg to a new model which would have a roll-on sleeve incorporating a pin which anchors the leg in the prosthetic. Also, the foot would have flexibility, as in bending symmetrically, as you walk. On 2nd June, 2015 a cast was taken for the new leg, and on the 23rd June at Prostek, my Prosthetist, Bridie, fitted the new prosthetic.

The prosthetics I had had to date looked like a piece of pipe with a foot fitted at the bottom, however, on 3rd August, 2015 my Prosthetist fitted a natural looking cover over the pipe. Some amputees are happy with just the pipe, but I find there is less scrutiny or attention drawn to me with having my pipe covered and appearing more natural.

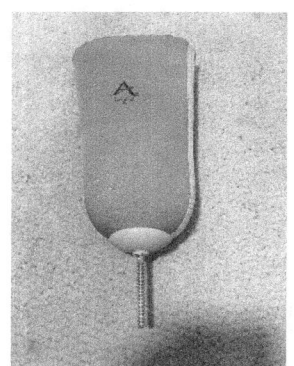
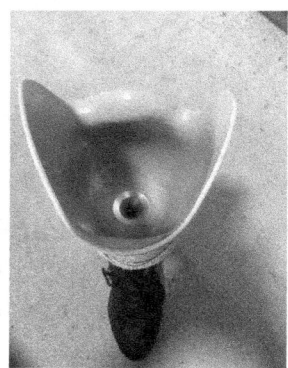

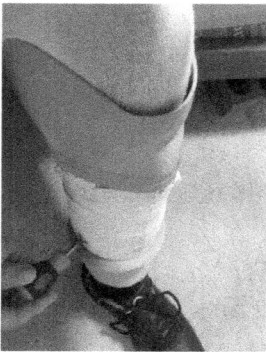

At this point in time I was managing to walk reasonably well, and I became a volunteer for Meals On Wheels, which I enjoyed and also kept me fit, whilst giving me practice and experience with my prosthetic leg.

In December 2015 I was preparing to go out, and in my haste, as I went to turn around my prosthetic foot stuck on the floor (as you have no feeling, you only think you have lifted it). I fell, but as I fell I twisted my (prosthetic leg) knee badly. So back to the Queen Elizabeth Hospital Emergency department in my wheelchair, where I had an x-ray and an ultra-sound. Everything was fine, just torn ligaments, so I spent the next two weeks in my wheelchair until they healed, and I could manage my prosthetic again.

At this stage I gave away volunteering, as I felt I was not confident enough carrying hot meals and soup, because if I tripped or fell I may have hurt a customer.

Throughout the summer of 2016 I set myself a task of walking 2 kilometres each day. I quite often went to the beach, which kept me fit and healthy but come winter I walked very little, as I did not want to go out in the cold and catch the flu'.

In May 2016, my stump had shrunk and so Prostek took another cast, and made a new socket to fit to my existing prosthetic. A different type of pin was also fitted where a screw driver is able to wind the stump into the socket, thus giving a much firmer fit.

As time went on I was finding I could not walk very far at all due to like a tightness or lack of sensation. Normally the stump felt fine, but now to the touch felt really cold. My Prosthetic Physician referred me to have an ultrasound then to visit a Vascular Specialist, and all showed to be in order. The Vascular Specialist concluded it was most likely 'Phantom pain' and that I should take my medication, "Lyrica/Pregablin 25mg, twice a day".

I have always had the medication, but I would only take it when I got, what I knew as Phantom pain. This is extreme pain which comes from nowhere and strikes like a lightning bolt; fortunately, I don't get this pain very often.

I was advised this medication is meant to be taken continuously, unlike the way I was taking it. However, this did not help my problem of the sensation of tightness I was getting, so I stopped taking the medication. Like many medications, especially painkillers, there may be side effects, one of which is constipation.

Upon examining my stump, I found it was tender at the end of the bone, so I cut up a gel sock to make a round gel double thickness buffer on the end of my stump. I experimented with different ways of fitting the prosthetic, for example with different types of socks, still firm but not feeling tight, and found I could walk much better and further without pain or discomfort.

Summary of Prosthetic

Obviously, a Prosthetic is something new and unfamiliar which was forced on me, however I accepted the challenge. Yes, it has been a rollercoaster of a ride, but nothing as cruel as Cancer and the Chemo treatment.

The Prosthetist cannot understand all that you are going through, and you cannot live on their doorstep, so it's up to the individual to find ways to help make it work, by experimenting and finding variations to help yourself.

Chapter 11

My Recovery after Hospital

Upon leaving hospital, I was still having Chemotherapy treatment. Once this treatment had finished I underwent the fitting and learning to walk on my prosthetic, as also previously documented.

From late in 2014, with all this in the past, I was on the road to getting back to everyday life where I took every day as it came. I enjoy cooking, and had good meals, gradually gaining the weight I had lost. I am lucky enough to have a car so I have been able to get out and about like going to the beach for walks.

It is now mid-February 2017 and I am thankfully still in remission. I am still walking fine but the prosthetic is always a challenge, yet so much better than a wheelchair.

I have been writing this story over the past year and there have been difficult and emotional times especially; when writing the chapters on chemotherapy, and reading the files when sifting through my pile of Hospital Records. Clare Hospital, ninety A4 Pages; Lyell McEwen, one hundred and seventy-seven A4 pages and Queen Elizabeth Hospital, one thousand three hundred and twenty A4 pages, as well my personal text records.

Summary

Thank you for reading this story of my Non-Hodgkin T-Cell Lymphoma and amputation of my leg.

I hope this true story, and the facts and details within, help others to persevere and cope and learn how you can help yourself.

Kind Regards to All,

Trevor A Harris

Appendix A: Thankyou

I thank all the medical people whom performed to a high professional standard; that is from all the five hospitals, plus Prostek, RDNS and all the clinics and surgeries involved whom attended me along the way. The Vascular Surgeons, my Haematologist, Doctor James, my home chemotherapy services Oncology Nurse Vinnie, my Clinical Psychologist Sarah, my Specialist Rehabilitation (Prosthetic) Physician Adrian, my Director of Physiotherapy Melisa, my Physiotherapist David, my GP Doctor Fong, plus my Prosthetist Professionals Bridie and Steve from "Prostek", and to anyone whom I may have forgotten to mention. I also thank all my family and friends, whom all showed care, and gave me hope and encouragement. Especially those who came and looked after me at home whilst I was undergoing chemotherapy treatment; my son Kevin, his wife Jane and family, my daughter Donna and husband Peter and family, my Brother Rex, Gail (my wife from whom I am separated), and Gail's daughter Lisa, Christine Davies (publishing advisor) Plus Vickie Collister (Nurse Medical advisor/editor) for spending many hours of her time assisting me.

Finally, I specially thank Wendy Egan who spent many hours of her own time and edited this book for me and assisted me with this project, thus enabling the publication of this book.

Appendix B: About myself

I was born in New Zealand on the 3rd September 1939, on the day that World War II was declared. I am a "Kiwi" with a dry sense of humour, and a sun-lover.

I have lived in Adelaide, South Australia, since February 1999, after moving from New Zealand, and became an Australian Citizen in 2002. Therefore, I have Dual Citizenship for Australia and New Zealand, and I have lived on my own since my wife and I separated in 2012.

The following are photos of me before and after my operations.

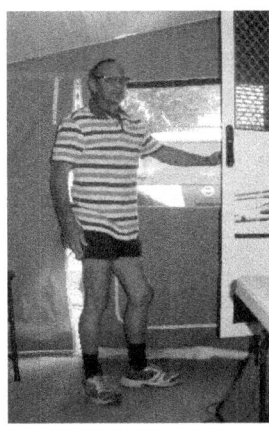
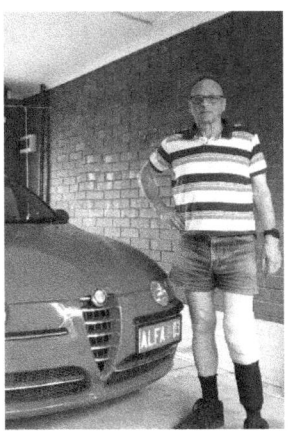

Before amputation *After amputation*

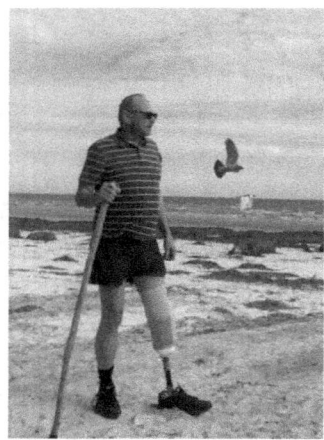 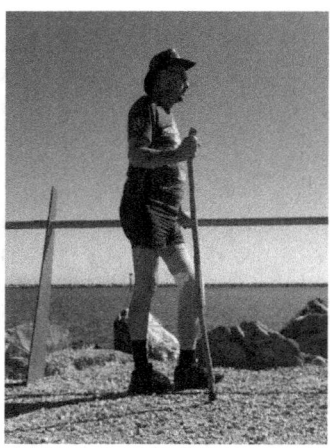

On the Beach   *At the Harbour*

I am a retired businessman, in the field of Industrial Electrical/Electronics/PLC/Computers/AutoCAD Drafting.

In 1960 I completed an Electrical apprenticeship and have spent my life in the Electrical/Electronics' Trade and still hold a South Australian "A Grade" Electrical Licence.

My sporting interests areV8 Motor Racing, Tennis, Rugby, Netball and AFL; in the past I also enjoyed boating and fishing.

My general interests are driving in my Alfa Romeo, cooking, and computing (for example, building and configuring computers plus creating websites).

I often drove to the beach, where I sat and recorded this story on my iPhone 6s+.

From February 1999, I worked full time at a Malt Factory in Port Adelaide, as a Maintenance Electrician and AutoCAD Draftsman. In 2004 (at the age of 65) I reduced my hours to twenty (20) hours per week, mainly doing AutoCAD drawing. Then, I finally retired in 2010, at the age of 71.

In 2012 I purchased a 2007 Four-wheel drive Nissan Navara, and a 2007 Caravan. I also purchased a half acre block of land, with several mature trees, backing onto farmland in the small town of Brinkworth, South Australia, as a base for travel around Australia.

I did a trip North to Whyalla (South Australia), plus other small local trips. Another trip I made was following the Murray River over to NSW and Victoria, then back up the coast via Robe to Adelaide.

On the half acre block, at Brinkworth I built new fences and decided to install power and water. Being an Electrician, I did all this myself late in 2013, and early 2014. I also planted trees along with self-watering systems.

I was 74 years old, and managing to dig ditches, lay cables and pipes, and build and install the electrical switch board, for the electrical and plumbing Installations.

To summarize, I was fit and well and living a normal life until struck by this disease.

About Writing this Story

In order to write my story, and to aid my memory of events, I obtained my Medical Records from the five hospitals which included:

- Clare Hospital Records 66xA4 pages
- Lyell McEwin Hospital Records 177xA4 pages.
- Queen Elizabeth combined with RAH plus St Margaret Hospital Records total 1,317xA4 pages

as in the photo below.

Thus, for the entire thirteen weeks in four hospitals I had a grand total of 1,560 A4 pages of paper records. I also received these records in PDF format which allowed me easier access to the files. Additionally, I downloaded my texts from my iPhone for this period, and printed them out.

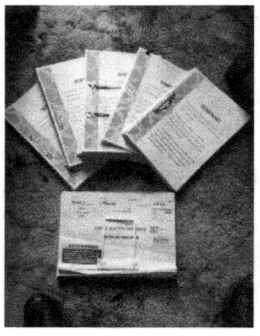

Most days I drove to the beach in my small Alfa Romeo and sat dictating into my iPhone 6sPlus, while reading from my texts (recorded over the period of my sickness) and Hospital records, to jog my memory of events.

The iPhone recording was automatically transformed to text and emailed to my home computer, where I transferred it to Word and edited the story. I have added all the texts between myself and my son over this period, at the end of this story, as authentication of the story.

All this took its toll on me and I became upset many times due to reliving the journey over and over, but I would just take a break for a day, as I did want to complete this story.

Appendix C: About Lymphoma

Lymphoma is the general term for cancers that develop in the lymphatic system. The lymphatic system is made up of a vast network of vessels (similar to blood vessels) that branch out into all the tissues of the body. These vessels contain lymph, a colorless watery fluid that carries lymphocytes, which are specialized white blood cells that fight infection. There are two types of lymphocytes, B-lymphocytes and T-lymphocytes (also called B-cells and T-cells). These cells protect us by making antibodies and destroying harmful microorganisms such as bacteria and viruses.

Lymphoma originates in developing B-lymphocytes and T-lymphocytes, which have undergone a malignant change. This means that they multiply without any proper order, forming tumors which are collections of cancer cells. These tumors cause swelling in the lymph nodes and other parts of the body.

Over time, malignant lymphocytes (called lymphoma cells) crowd out normal lymphocytes and eventually the immune system becomes weakened and can no longer function properly. Significant advances are continually being made in the way your lymphoma can be managed. This means that with treatment, many people can now be cured. Many others who are treated remain disease-free and well for a long time.

Sub-types of Lymphoma

There are more than 40 different sub-types of lymphoma currently recognized by the World Health Organization's classification system.

Five of these sub-types belong to a group of diseases called Hodgkin lymphoma. All other sub-types are commonly grouped together and called non-Hodgkin lymphomas.

How common is non-Hodgkin Lymphoma?

Each year in Australia around 4000 people are diagnosed with a type of B-cell or T-cell lymphoma making them the most common type of blood cancer diagnosed. Overall, they represent the sixth most common type of cancer in men, and the fifth most common type of cancer in women.

Who gets non-Hodgkin Lymphoma?

Lymphomas can occur at any age but they are more common in adults over the age of 50. Lymphomas occur more frequently in men than in women. In children, non-Hodgkin lymphoma and leukemia are some of the most common types of cancer seen, but this number is far fewer than in the adult population. Lymphomas in children tend to grow quickly and they are often curable.

What Causes non-Hodgkin Lymphoma?

In most cases the exact cause of lymphoma remains unknown, but they are thought to result from damage to one or more of the genes that normally control the development of blood cells. Research is going on all the time into possible causes of this damage. In most cases people who are diagnosed with lymphoma have no family history of the disease. Like many cancers, damage to special proteins that control the growth and division of cells may play a role in the development of lymphoma.

The following are factors which may put some people at a higher risk of developing lymphoma:

- immunosuppression – a small percentage of lymphomas occur in people whose immune system has been weakened either by a viral infection or as a result of drugs that affect the function of the immune system

- infection – particularly in people with immunosuppression, viruses such as the Epstein-Barr virus or the human T-cell leukemia/lymphoma virus may damage developing lymphocytes

- chemicals – some evidence suggest that people exposed to high concentrations of agricultural chemicals may have a higher risk of developing lymphoma

- lifestyle – lifestyle factors including smoking and obesity can increase the risk of developing lymphoma.

What are the symptoms of non-Hodgkin Lymphoma?
Some people do not have any symptoms when they are first diagnosed with lymphoma. In these cases the disease

may be picked up by accident, for example during a routine chest x-ray. Lymphoma commonly presents as a firm, usually painless swelling of a lymph node (swollen glands), usually in the neck, under the arms or in the groin.

It is important to remember that most people who go to their doctor with enlarged lymph nodes do not have lymphoma. Swollen glands often result from an infection, for example a sore throat. In this case the glands in the neck are usually swollen and painful.

Other symptoms may include:

- regular and frequent fevers
- excessive sweating, usually at night
- unintentional weight loss
- persistent fatigue and lack of energy
- generalized itching

Sometimes lymphoma starts in the lymph nodes in deeper parts of the body like those found in the abdomen (causing bloating), or the lymph nodes in the chest (causing coughing, discomfort in the chest and difficulty breathing). When it is first diagnosed, it is common for lymphoma to be found in several different sites in the body at once. It can spread to any organ and may involve the spleen, liver, brain and spinal cord (central nervous system) and bone marrow.

Some of these symptoms may also be seen in other illnesses, including viral infections. It is important to see your doctor if you have any symptoms that do not go away so that you can be examined and treated properly.

Appendix D: About Amputation

Amputation is an irreversible change, the loss of a part of the body is one of the most invasive interventions in the body that one can experience. No matter if it is an arm or a leg to be amputated, it is never easy, however it may be a bit easier if one accepts help and advice.

Reasons for amputation

There are different causes that can lead to amputation. It is essential whether the person can prepare for years during an illness before the amputation, or whether the loss of a limb is caused by a traumatic event.

The most common reason for amputation of the lower extremities are vascular diseases. Other causes are, for example, diabetes, accidents or cancer. Amputations of the upper extremities are about 17 times rarer. The most common cause is trauma.

Amputations worldwide are significantly increasing due to the increase of disorders like diabetes mellitus and arterial occlusive diseases. If someone has the chance to prepare for an amputation, this time before the operation should be used as efficiently as possible so that the healing and rehabilitation can optimally process.

It is important to take into account both the physical and the psychological aspects that arise with a medical intervention. It is important to be informed early by the attending physician about the process and the consequences of the surgery. All questions about the surgical procedure, the treatment and possible prosthesis should be answered and any uncertainties relating to business and private life clarified.

Relatives should be involved in the entire process of the amputation. They are very important and can actively support the patient both morally and practically.

As an additional source of information and support, other people with amputations may be consulted. Fear, anxiety and uncertainty can be reduced by the personal experiences of people with amputations. However, it must be clear that the treatment process is individual and direct comparisons with other patients are not possible.

Finding the right attitude to amputation

An important point is the personal attitude of the patient towards the amputation. The amputation should be viewed as a positive step towards improvement or stabilization of health. The recovery and rehabilitation can only be successful if the patient is actively involved in the entire process.

The before and after

Patients often feel anxious before an amputation and sometimes very depressed. For many patients, the imagination is worse than the reality, and they quickly learn to cope with the new situation surprisingly well. Other people need a little more time and can, for example, not yet look at the stump at the beginning during changing the dressing. With patience and affection, the patient can usually accept his condition soon. It is important that we and the relatives can accept the patient as a full person; this transfers to the patient and his/her self-esteem.

The time between surgery and prosthetic adjustment

For most affected people, the process between surgery and adjustment of prostheses is particularly exhausting and tedious.

Affected people face a variety of changes after the amputation. In addition to the physical function limitations, developments in the psychosocial field play a crucial role. Often, changes in professional and family environment have to be processed.

In this phase, many specialists are working together to ensure the most possible mobility and flexibility for the patient. In addition to these physical activities, the psychological rehabilitation and social situation also play essential roles.

The majority of amputee's experiences stump pains or phantom pains during this phase. Stump pains are caused by processes that are localized in the stump itself. Phantom pains can occur after the removal or denervation of a limb. They take on different pain characteristics and are triggered by various factors. Phantom sensations are sensations in the area of the no longer existing limbs.

There is no formula for coping with an amputation.

Appendix E: About Lyrica/Pregabalin

Lyrica is a brand name for the drug Pregabalin and is often prescribed to Amputees for Phantom pain and it should only be used as Directed by your Medical Physician or Chemist.

Appendix F: Reports by Haematologist

Before starting my Chemotherapy treatment, the Haematologist outlined the treatment to me and my son. The treatment was to be six rounds of Chemotherapy increasing the dosage, from and including round four, by twenty percent.

He then advised that every three months to six months he would arrange for me to have blood tests, followed by an appointment to examine and report on my progress. At these appointments, he would physically examine me plus show and explain the results of my blood tests.

In summing up he always stated:
'**There is no cure for non-Hodgkin's Lymphoma** and that it is very aggressive.' He also went on to say if the Lymphoma returns it will be difficult to treat as he had already administered the strongest dosage of Chemotherapy that he could administer safely, implying that any further treatment would only be effective if a stronger than the previous treatment is available to administer safely.

The advice was "Just go and live Normally"

Report by Haematologist, 7 November, 2014
Re: Trevor HARRIS DOB: 3.9.39

Diagnosis: Angioimmunoblastic T-cell NHL

Treatment: DA-EPOCH x six cycles, completed September 2014

Peripheral vascular disease

Venous thromboembolic disease, left cephalic vein, by non-occluive thrombus

Left below knee amputee

Asbestosis

Hypertension Current medications: Clexane 40 mg daily, Aspirin 100 mg daily, Gabapentin 50 mg daily, Pantoprazole 40 mg daily

Mr. Trevor Harris, accompanied by his son, was reviewed in the Outpatient Clinic at TQEH. As you know, Trevor is 75 years of age, diagnosed with angioimmunoblastic T-cell lymphoma in April 2014. His presentation was complicated by acute ischaemia of left leg and angiography revealed critical, 90%, stenosis at the left common femoral artery. Endarterectomy with thrombectomy was unsuccessful and embolisation resulted in full occlusion of distal artery on the left side. Trevor underwent a below knee amputation in April 2014. Staging of T-cell lymphoma by CT and PET, revealed widespread disseminated lymphadenopathy. Bone marrow biopsy revealed lymphoma infiltration. In addition, Trevor has a past history of asbestos exposure and plaques were noted on the pleura at CT scan. Trevor was treated with dose adjusted EPOCH (etoposide, prednisone, vincristine, cyclophosphamide and doxorubicin). This was complicated by venous thrombosis of the left cephalic vein. Ultimately Trevor received six cycles of dose adjusted EPOCH, which was completed in September 2014.

On review today, Trevor is again in good spirits and self-mobilising in a wheelchair or prosthetic limb. He now lives at home and is managing well. He has completed six cycles of dose adjusted EPOCH in September 2014. Available blood cell indices are four weeks old and show Hb 109, WCC 8.26 and platelets 149. The yGT is mildly elevated at 106 with alk phos at 150. LOH is 301. Post treatment CT scan show a very good response with some small residual nodes in the areas that were previously enlarged. PET scan shows no evidence of FOG avidity.

Trevor has completed treatment and is currently in complete remission. I have ceased the prophylactic Famciclovir, Fluconazole and Bactrim. I plan to review him in three months

Report by Haematologist, 8 April, 2016

Re: Trevor HARRIS   DOB: 3.9.39

Diagnosis: Angioimmunoblastic T-cell NHL

Treatment: DA-EPOCH x six cycles, completed September:2014

Peripheral vascular disease Venous thromboembolic disease, left cephalic vein, by non-occlusive thrombus

Left below knee amputee

Asbestosis

Hypertension

Current medications: Pregabalin, PRN (phantom pain), Aspirin

Mr. Trevor Harris, accompanied by his son, was reviewed in the outpatient clinic at TQEH. As you know, Trevor is 76 years of age, diagnosed with angioimmunoblastic T-cell lymphoma in April 2014. His presentation was complicated by acute ischaemia of left leg and angiography revealed critical, 90%, stenosis at the left common femoral artery. Endarterectomy with thrombectomy was unsuccessful and embolisation resulted in full occlusion of distal artery on the left side. Trevor underwent a below knee amputation in April 2014. Staging of T-cell lymphoma by CT and PET, revealed widespread disseminated lymphadenopathy. Bone marrow biopsy revealed lymphoma infiltration. In addition, Trevor has a past history of asbestos exposure and plaques were noted on the pleura at CT scan. Trevor was treated with dose adjusted EPOCH (etoposide, prednisone, vincristine, cyclophosphamide and doxorubicin). This was complicated by venous thrombosis of the left cephalic vein. Ultimately Trevor received six cycles of dose adjusted EPOCH, which was completed in September 2014.

On review today, Trevor describes a fall that he had in December which left him wheelchair bound for a while, but he is now ambulating on his prosthetic limb, using a hiking stick for additional support. Trevor otherwise feels well. Because of the falls risk, he no longer works for "Meals on Wheels", which I can tell disappoints him. There is no lymphadEJnopathy on physical exam and abdominal examination is unremarkable. Mild LFT abnormalities persist, but are stable. LOH is only mildly elevated at 302 and also stable. Renal function shows an eGFR of 74 ml/min and remaining electrolytes are normal. Blood cell indices show Hb 160, wee 5.5 and platelets 143. There 1s no immun,e-paresis, as IgG fraction measures 5.8 g/L.

In summary, Trevor remains in complete remission and I have made no changes to current management. I plan to continue bi-annual surveillance, keeping you informed of developments.

Appendix G: Clinical Report: 24/04/2014

CT ANGIOGRAM AORTO BIFEMORAL

CLINICAL DETAILS: Ischaemic left foot weaker femoral and popliteal pulse. No dorsalis pedis/popli teal .

TECHNIQUE: Arterial imaging of the abdominal aorta and lower limb arteries performed.

REPORT: Additional clinical history of T cell lymphoma noted.

There is calcification of the abdominal aorta which is non aneurysmal. There is no stenosis seen involving the aorta or its anterior branches. The renal arteries are widely patent.

The common iliac arteries show further evidence of calcified plaque. There is a 50% stenosis secondary to calcific plaque at the origin of the left common iliac artery. No external or internal iliac artery stenosis detected.

LEFT LEG: Densely calcified plaque causes a 90% stenosis of the proximal common femoral artery. This results in significant delay and contrast opacification beyond this vessel although it still is seen to remain patent.

The superficial femoral and popliteal arteries are widely patent with no significant atheromatous disease.

Multi focal occlusive disease involves the anterior tibial artery through its length and there is an occlusion of the posterior tibial artery at the mid-calf level. The peroneal artery is occluded close to its origin. There is reconstitution of flow via collaterals seen in the distal anterior tibial artery at the ankle levels.

RIGHT LEG: Eccentric calcified plaque involves the CFA without significant stenosis. The SFA popliteal arteries are widely patent.

There is three vessel runoff to the ankle identified although visualisation of the vessels at the ankle level are somewhat limited by metallic artefact from a distal fibular plate and screw fixator.

Findings discussed without formal reconstruction.

OTHER FINDINGS: There is gross splenomegaly in numerous retroperitoneal lymph nodes consistent with the additional history of lymphoma.

A right basal pleural effusion with associated atel ectasi s/consoli dati on identified. A small left effusion is seen. Multiple calcified pleural plaques are identified. The pancreas, visualised portion of the liver, adrenals and kidneys appear normal. There are multiple mesenteric lymph nodes seen.

The gallbladder is contracted. There is an impression of mild gallbladder wall thickening although assessment is limited due to lack of distention.

There is a small amount of free fluid noted in the paracolic gutters bilaterally.

COMMENT: There is a critical stenosis measuring > 90% secondary to calcified plaque at the proximal left CFA level.

Through the left calf arteries show multifocal disease and are occluded throughout. There is reconstitution of flow suspected within the distal ATA likely via collateral.

Findings were discussed with the referring vascular clinicians at the time of scanning.

Amputation Record: 26/04/2014

LEFT BELOW KNEE EMBOLECTOMY ALI L. limb - threatened GA. IVABx. IDC. Art line.
General Anaesthetic
LEFT BELOW KNEE EMBOLECTOMY ALI L. limb - threatened GA. IVABx. IDC. Art line.
Medial approach to L. BK popliteal artery - soleal arch taken down - mod oedematous but healthy muscle Ant. tibial v. divided and ligated with 3.0 vicryl

ATA/PTA/PA all dissected out and controlled Heparin 3000U given - prev. IV heparin infusion

Transverse arteriotomy of TPT - snall branch origin used for PA access SFA inflow re-evaluated + cleared of thrombus

3F fogharty thrombectomy of ATA to below ankle - long mixed clot extracted with low-resistence flush post - clot sent for Thrombectomy of PA/PTA - Good length of clot extracted from both bt unable to pass catheter to below ankle level in PTA 240 mcg GTN given / 100000U urokinase to tibials

Both arteriotomies closed with 6.0/7.0 prolene Haemostasis

Completion II runs - good flow in ATA to plantar arch - sluggish PA/PTA flow not crossing ankle Closed in layers with vicryl / monocryl - 10F drain in + secured To HDU

Appendix H: Report by Psychologist

26 May 2015

Re: Trevor HARRIS DOB: 03.09.1939

I am writing to provide an update of Trevor's involvement with our clinical psychology service. As you will recall, I have been providing psychological support to Trevor through our outpatient clinic for assistance with improving his mood and adjustment to his diagnosis of T-Cell Lymphoma.

Since his referral to our service in July 2014, I have seen Trevor for six psychology appointments. During these appointments, I have provided Trevor with supportive counselling, psychoeducation, and introduced to him cognitive behavioural therapy strategies for improving his mood. These strategies included behaviour activation (scheduling daily activities that create pleasure and/or a sense of achievement) as well as increasing his engagement in activities that provide him with a sense of purpose. We also discussed acknowledged) the positive impact of engaging socially with family members and friends.

In addition to this I have provided Trevor with psychoeducation about emotions and coping strategies for him to utilise at times of emotional distress, particularly when he is feeling worried regarding his cancer returning. In doing so, I have also validated the distress he has experienced given the significant impact his cancer has had on his lifestyle and wellbeing. Trevor has responded well to such interventions and reports that his mood and coping abilities have improved.

Appendix I: Report by Rehabilitation Physician 13 April, 2015

Trevor was seen in the Amputee Clinic on 13th April, 2015. He is wearing an interim prosthesis which is fitting reasonably well with a silicone sock and a silicone suspension sleeve. Trevor's stump volume is stabilized. He occasionally has some tenderness over the distal aspect of his fibula remnant but he was not tender in this area today.

Trevor is going overseas for a trip to New Zealand for 2 weeks later this month.

I have raised a prescription for a definitive prosthesis for him and this will be fabricated on his return. The prosthesis will be a Patella Tendon Bearing prosthesis with a silicone sleeve suspension.

Trevor continues on Pregabalin 25 mg 2 tablets twice daily and I will provide him with a prescription to cover him until his next review.

Appendix J: My Story by Text

(SMS) Transcripts

The following is my journey told by text messages recorded between my son and myself, which reads almost as a running commentary.

Prelude: I Had been sick for two or three days, Coughing, Hot Sweats, Chills, Vomiting, Sore Chest, Shaking all over uncontrollably, and with swollen feet from time to time.

Insert: At Home in Brinkworth.

[Friday, 28 March 2014 12:43:29 PM] Me: Very sick rang Doc in Two Wells as had Apt re results blood tests but too sick he called ambo for me, now admitted Clare hosp

Insert: Clare Hospital.

[Friday, 28 March 2014 1:24:56 PM] Kevin: Prob a good thing for you to help get through problems faster. Let me know what action that take and how things are going later if possible

[Friday, 28 March 2014 1:50:14 PM] Me: Doctor just been says its still chest problem more antibiotics

[Saturday, 29 March 2014 6:57:02 PM] Kevin: Any news from Dr?

[Saturday, 29 March 2014 7:37:06 PM] Me: Doctor been said have to wait for antibiotics to do the job said have to drink heaps, Am drinking ok at moment i am stuffed!

[Sunday, 30 March 2014 10:40:40 AM] Kevin: How was last night?

[Sunday, 30 March 2014 10:44:12 AM] Me: Two bed changes shakes as well but feeling better today

[Sunday, 30 March 2014 1:59:41 PM] Kevin: Hopefully your still on the rise Is Doctor expected back again today?

[Monday, 31 March 2014 10:55:05 AM] Kevin: How was your night, feeling any better today?

[Monday, 31 March 2014 2:57:23 PM] Me: Got kicked out at 11 am had good night but nothing like ok! friend's bought me home

Insert: Back at Home in Brinkworth.

[Tuesday, 1 April 2014 6:25:17 AM] Me: Had a reasonable night, had 2 slices of ham and half plate peaches yesterday and still there far from right going see if can get a C pillow as i need to be elevated all the time also thermometer to check my temp

[Tuesday, 1 April 2014 8:07:04 AM] Kevin: Glad to hear your nights getting better but if things go downhill even a little bit head straight back to hospital or else you will be back to where you were last week.

[Tuesday, 1 April 2014 1:48:06 PM] Me: My temp was 38deg is now 37.5 deg i like to keep track of it had two slices of ham

[Wednesday, 2 April 2014 7:32:31 AM] Kevin: Good to hear and hopefully cooler days and nights will help. Keep track if temp, 37.5 sounds better but if starts to rise get help

[Thursday, 3 April 2014 9:47:12 AM] Kevin: Seems it's just not moving from chest. Keep antibiotics going until well and truly gone. Are you still eating at least a little bit each day?

[Friday, 4 April 2014 2:44:23 PM] Kevin: Good to hear things getting better now need to get eating back in order.

[Friday, 4 April 2014 2:56:30 PM] Me: going doc shortly

[Friday, 4 April 2014 5:29:44 PM] Me: stuffed up appointment with Dr mon not frid after driving there now have swollen feet

[Saturday, 5 April 2014 9:25:33 AM] Me: Two lots of overnight sweats feet less swollen temp down for first time to 36.5 been in high 37s

[Sunday, 6 April 2014 2:07:20 PM] Kevin: How you feeling today, any better than this time last week?!!

[Sunday, 6 April 2014 2:14:16 PM] Me: Still up and down had big sweat overnight temp went sky high today 39.1!!! have laid under air con got temp down to 37.8 felt ok yesterday and had some tea today have that unsettled tummy, just going round and round

[Sunday, 6 April 2014 2:15:08 PM] Kevin: Back to dr tomorrow? Still taking antibiotics?

[Sunday, 6 April 2014 2:15:29 PM] Me: yes

[Monday, 7 April 2014 7:01:41 PM] Me: Going back hospital 9am

[Monday, 7 April 2014 7:01:44 PM] Kevin: Has dr told you to go? Are you worse again?

[Tuesday, 8 April 2014 12:12:08 PM] Kevin: Are you back in hospital, what's the latest?

[Tuesday, 8 April 2014 12:18:43 PM] Me: Dr never organized hospital so still home???

[Tuesday, 8 April 2014 4:31:27 PM] Kevin: What's next then, Dr calling them or do you need to just go there yourself if still not right

[Tuesday, 8 April 2014 4:43:08 PM] Me: Doc rang being admitted 7pm

[Tuesday, 8 April 2014 4:43:04 PM] Kevin: Is Gail taking you there tonight?

[Tuesday, 8 April 2014 4:44:22 PM] Me: yes

[Tuesday, 8 April 2014 4:45:12 PM] Kevin: Ok let me know once there and what the action is

[Tuesday, 8 April 2014 4:46:55 PM] Me: let you know in morning

Insert: Back in Clare Hospital.
[Tuesday, 8 April 2014 9:03:32 PM] Me: finally in hospital on drip 9pm

[Tuesday, 8 April 2014 9:31:04 PM] Kevin: Good to hear, hope you have good night. Talk tomorrow

[Wednesday, 9 April 2014 6:52:39 AM] Me: Had bad night, in a way is good as they know what i am up against the nurse said i should of been here days ago!

[Wednesday, 9 April 2014 10:44:40 AM] Kevin: Why are it nights worse than day, seems strange do you notice more at night cause can't sleep?

[Wednesday, 9 April 2014 1:36:25 PM] Me: Dr been more tests tomorrow just a waiting game

[Wednesday, 9 April 2014 9:26:02 PM] Me: Been bad, transferring lyell McEwin in about an hr for specialist

[Wednesday, 9 April 2014 9:33:12 PM] Kevin Harris: Ok, not good. Let me know when you get there. Don't worry about time.

Insert: Lyell McEwin Hospital.

[Thursday, 10 April 2014 6:50:00 AM] Kevin Did you check in to Lyle Mac ok, when will you see spec?

[Thursday, 10 April 2014 6:50:19 AM] Me: Arrived lyell Mc 12.30am still in emergency but are admitting me. Had bad turn 10 pm in Clare Dr was there sent me here had bad turn here 5am 2x Drs 3 nurses!!

[Thursday, 10 April 2014 6:54:16 AM] Kevin : Ok can come there after work.

[Thursday, 10 April 2014 6:58:06 AM] Me: I think could be here a while up to you but i am now needing support

[Thursday, 10 April 2014 7:25:57 AM] Kevin : Let me know when you are in a room and I will come there.

[Thursday, 10 April 2014 7:47:47 AM] Me: Would be best if you come now and talk doc at emergency

[Thursday, 10 April 2014 7:49:28 AM] Kevin: Ok no probs wasn't sure if I was allowed in emergency. Will do that, if you move let me know.

[Thursday, 10 April 2014 8:06:20 AM] Me: ok

[Thursday, 10 April 2014 8:23:48 AM] Me: emerg room 9

[Thursday, 10 April 2014 5:32:03 PM] Me: Been asleep woke up wet sweat had shower ok.

[[Thursday, 10 April 2014 6:29:41 PM] Me: Just eaten some tea hope it stays there have not seen Dr been big day may be best you come tomorow night

[Thursday, 10 April 2014 6:29:44 PM] Kevin: Ok let me know in morning how things are going. Hopefully Dr not far away.

[Thursday, 10 April 2014 6:31:05 PM] Me: ok

[Friday, 11 April 2014 6:47:35 AM] Me: Had a good night best for weeks not all plain sailing but ok dont worry coming today may have a list for you

[Friday, 11 April 2014 7:03:32 AM] Kevin: Glad to hear the night was a little better and hopefully caught up on some sleep. Have you seen Dr yet?

[Friday, 11 April 2014 10:00:37 AM] Me: Seen Dr got Ct scan 2.45pm thats all till results

 [Friday, 11 April 2014 4:42:40 PM] Me: went for Ct at 2pm just got back

 [Friday, 11 April 2014 4:59:50 PM] Me: The scans will have to go to spec Dr then to Dr then he will see what ever however this morn he checked my glands armpits and he said swollen! hope to eat some tea feeling stuffed after all that

 [Saturday, 12 April 2014 9:00:51 AM] Me: Night ok till 4am woke up sweat had shower new sheets then 7am got shivers had *panadol came right was hot about midnight so Dr came took blood!!! aint got much left.*

[Saturday, 12 April 2014 9:08:11 AM] Kevin: More blood!

[Saturday, 12 April 2014 9:09:06 PM] Me: The regular team back on tonight makes it comforting they are all like family

[Sunday, 13 April 2014 7:22:19 AM] Me: normal night shivers sweats hot had shower 5am sitting at window in sun

[Sunday, 13 April 2014 9:19:18 AM] Me: Dr been only young one status wait till tomorrow

[Sunday, 13 April 2014 10:36:08 AM] Kevin: Ok, frustrating waiting for info but all in all seems a nice Hosp and staff so in good place and good hands as we see this thru.

[Monday, 14 April 2014 9:02:16 AM] Kevin: How was last night?

[Monday, 14 April 2014 9:10:55 AM] Me: Had very good night but have no energy

[Tuesday, 15 April 2014 6:59:04 AM] Me: Operation today!! dont know when was supposed to be told midnight just been told

[Tuesday, 15 April 2014 7:11:20 AM] Kevin Harris: Ok great at least things are happening. Did you have ok night?

[Tuesday, 15 April 2014 7:14:50 AM] Me: Night ok except coughed a lot

[Tuesday, 15 April 2014 9:20:31 AM] Me: Had visit by surgeons, I was impressed, it will be late morning.

[Tuesday, 15 April 2014 9:21:28 AM] Kevin: Ok all good. Take care

[Wednesday, 16 April 2014 6:48:35 AM] Me: Had good night await results?

[Wednesday, 16 April 2014 7:12:37 AM] Kevin: Glad nights are better. Will come out tonight after work.

[Wednesday, 16 April 2014 8:52:07 AM] Me: Surgeons been check said took two lumps out under arm results will be some days

ADDED detail: 16 April 2014 Sent home from Hospital to await Results
ADDED detail: Now in a Motel

[Thursday, 17 April 2014 6:32:56 AM] Kevin: You ok there in the Motel, was night all right?

[Sunday, 20 April 2014 8:58:26 AM] Me: Bad night need help washing good laundry here i am stuffed

ADDED detail: Very Sick so taken back to Lyell McEwin Hospital 20th April.

[Monday, 21 April 2014 6:57:34 AM] Me: Reasonable night waiting breakfast dont rush here will keep u up-to-date

[Monday, 21 April 2014 6:59:54 AM] Kevin: Good to hear

[Monday, 21 April 2014 9:40:40 AM] Kevin: Hope you are comfortable.

[Monday, 21 April 2014 9:44:44 AM] Me: I am ok no need come till later had shave shower removing Catheter shortly

[Monday, 21 April 2014 12:34:20 PM] Me: Now in room 13

[Monday, 21 April 2014 4:40:44 PM] Me: Nurse just told me i can have Panadol anytime and i should of been given last night!!!!!

[Monday, 21 April 2014 4:58:00 PM] Kevin: Great news, I had a word to her on way out!

[Tuesday, 22 April 2014 8:29:22 AM] Me: Good night no chills!!!

[Tuesday, 22 April 2014 8:32:24 AM] Kevin: Good to hear about night. [Tuesday, 22 April 2014 8:36:09 AM] Me: ok

[Tuesday, 22 April 2014 1:02:36 PM] Kevin: Still in same Hospital?

[Tuesday, 22 April 2014 1:03:53 PM] Me: Yeh they said could be late as still no confirmation

[Tuesday, 22 April 2014 3:34:37 PM] Me: Did nurse ring you regards going QE shortly??

[Tuesday, 22 April 2014 3:38:46 PM] Kevin: Yes all good and great news

ADDED detail: Now in Queen Elizabeth Hospital
[Tuesday, 22 April 2014 4:38:56 PM] Me: I am at QE

[Tuesday, 22 April 2014 4:40:56 PM] Kevin Harris: Ok let me know when in a ward bed with number etc

[Tuesday, 22 April 2014 5:58:59 PM] Me: NE ground B hematology room 23

[Tuesday, 22 April 2014 6:47:21 PM] Me: Can you get here by 7.30 i think they want talk to you

[Tuesday, 22 April 2014 6:53:12 PM] Kevin Harris: Ok coming now

[Wednesday, 23 April 2014 6:56:08 AM] Me: Had good night no chills no sweats! but not good sleep as foot sore all night can get pain relief tonight.

[Wednesday, 23 April 2014 7:09:12 AM] Kevin Harris : Great to hear about your night, yes foot looks sore. Will wait to hear from you

[Wednesday, 23 April 2014 7:16:29 AM] Me: Dont worry yep let you know soon as

[Wednesday, 23 April 2014 11:01:51 AM] Kevin Harris : Spoke to Dr while you were getting scan so don't worry too much if he sees you before I get back

[Wednesday, 23 April 2014 5:05:50 PM] Me: Just had foot x-rayed now waiting to go back!!!!!!!

[Wednesday, 23 April 2014 5:23:14 PM] Kevin Harris: Wow how many X-rays can you have!

[Wednesday, 23 April 2014 5:23:52 PM] Me: still waiting go back!!!!

[Wednesday, 23 April 2014 5:43:34 PM] Me: still!!!!

[Wednesday, 23 April 2014 6:13:45 PM] Me: just back in room stuffed

Insert: Went to the Royal Adelaide Hospital for a PET Scan

[Thursday, 24 April 2014 10:56:30 AM] Kevin Harris : Are you all good to leave for a RAH at 11-30?

[Thursday, 24 April 2014 11:23:10 AM] Me: yes ready now

[Thursday, 24 April 2014 12:52:10 PM] Me: will be about two hrs from now [Thursday, 24 April 2014 1:05:28 PM] Kevin Harris: What the hell for!!

[Thursday, 24 April 2014 2:55:25 PM] Me: I am ready

[Thursday, 24 April 2014 3:07:56 PM] Me: Sitting outside where you dropped me off

[Thursday, 24 April 2014 3:08:17 PM] Kevin Harris : Ok on way

Insert: Returned from the Royal Adelaide Hospital to the Queen Elizabeth Hospital

[Thursday, 24 April 2014 6:34:00 PM] Kevin Harris : Did you have foot scan or get seen by Dr about foot?

[Thursday, 24 April 2014 6:36:35 PM] Me: Doing it now and I am not happy she says not looking good now going do ultra sound

[Thursday, 24 April 2014 7:48:40 PM] Kevin Harris : Let me know what's happening with foot.

[Thursday, 24 April 2014 7:50:17 PM] Me: They going Op late tonight re clot

[Thursday, 24 April 2014 8:01:01 PM] Kevin Harris : Just tried to call Hospital and speak to them about it but no answer.

[Thursday, 24 April 2014 8:06:14 PM] Me: They spoke to Chemo boss they going fix clot in an hr then Chemo tomorrow

[Friday, 25 April 2014 10:03:17 AM] Me: Waiting on surgeons Cancer Dr men been waiting but all up to surgeon?

They want start Chemo but need me in ward so Surgeon Verse Chemo Dr

[Friday, 25 April 2014 10:06:16 AM] Kevin Harris :   Ok understand they want to start treatment ASAP.

[Friday, 25 April 2014 10:10:28 AM] Me: Until surgeon sees me and tells me stay in surgical ward or go Cancer ward thus surg v med they are in the building just waiting for them

[Friday, 25 April 2014 10:41:44 AM] Me: Cleared to go back to med ward!!

[Friday, 25 April 2014 10:42:29 AM] Kevin Harris : Ok let me know what room you end up in

[Friday, 25 April 2014 12:59:32 PM] Me: Just/still waiting on bed

[Friday, 25 April 2014 2:55:20 PM] Kevin Harris: You got new hotel room yet? They starting chemo today?

[Friday, 25 April 2014 2:56:16 PM] Me: Still waiting room!!!!!

[Friday, 25 April 2014 3:10:30 PM] Me: Just have bath in bed with drain from op catheter and drip!!!!!!!all hanging around

[Friday, 25 April 2014 3:41:12 PM] Kevin Harris: Sounds like fun! So you have new room no. Yet?

[Friday, 25 April 2014 3:44:11 PM] Me: No not yet feel good after bath

[Friday, 25 April 2014 4:13:50 PM] Me: On move dont know number yet

[Friday, 25 April 2014 4:35:28 PM] Me: Room 53

[Friday, 25 April 2014 4:36:40 PM] Kevin Harris: Welcome back! Will call round soon

[Friday, 25 April 2014 4:37:24 PM] Me: Back in room 53

[Saturday, 26 April 2014 6:31:57 AM] Me: After you went needed to go loo no one around so go myself there but when I put weight on foot had huge pain fell on floor nurse came. Consequently, had sore foot all night plus heaps pain killer otherwise ok

[Saturday, 26 April 2014 10:38:13 AM] Me: Operating again a few hrs ok

[Saturday, 26 April 2014 10:40:24 AM] Kevin Harris: Bloody hell. Problem with blood in leg still?

[Sunday, 27 April 2014 5:55:59 AM] Me: Surgeon was here at 4am hes not happy coming back in couple hrs looks like amputate

[Sunday, 27 April 2014 8:04:40 AM] Kevin Harris: Not good news but need to get leg sorted out so treatment can start. Spoke to your nurse an hour ago. Let me know if you want me to come there and see Surgeon or he can call me when he gets there.

[Sunday, 27 April 2014 8:09:04 AM] Me: Will let you know when he gets here

[Sunday, 27 April 2014 3:51:48 PM] Kevin Harris: Are you ok there?

[Sunday, 27 April 2014 3:53:21 PM] Me: All ok not come yet?

[Sunday, 27 April 2014 3:55:40 PM] Me: Now have my own press button pain relief!!!

[Sunday, 27 April 2014 3:56:08 PM] Kevin Harris: Remote control!

Insert: Foot Amputated overnight 27th April

[Monday, 28 April 2014 6:32:50 AM] Kevin Harris : How was night?

[Monday, 28 April 2014 7:22:14 AM] Me: Ok

[Monday, 28 April 2014 8:07:39 AM] Me: Ok, Drs + breakfast all go

[Monday, 28 April 2014 7:40:56 PM] Me: Drifting in and out

[Monday, 28 April 2014 7:42:09 PM] Kevin Harris : Will come back soon.

[Monday, 28 April 2014 7:55:22 PM] Me: Dont come back as they have emergency here

[Monday, 28 April 2014 8:05:37 PM] Kevin Harris : Ok spoke to nurse, all good. You keep chin up and don't worry about anything. Stay comfortable and pain free. We are all here if you need us get them to call.

[Wednesday, 30 April 2014 9:13:52 PM] Kevin Harris : Shall we come now or in the morning?

[Wednesday, 30 April 2014 9:19:12 PM] Me: Dont worry tonight

[Wednesday, 30 April 2014 9:20:07 PM] Kevin Harris: Just left will come for few mins

[Thursday, 1 May 2014 9:13:28 PM] Kevin Harris: Have day off tomorrow so will be at hospital. Hope all good there tonight and quiet for you.

[Friday, 2 May 2014 7:01:03 AM] Me: Night about same had wash etc

[Friday, 2 May 2014 7:50:08 AM] Me: No chemo yet

[Friday, 2 May 2014 11:35:59 AM] Me: Having Chemo today!!!

[Friday, 2 May 2014 12:08:58 PM] Kevin Harris :   Donna and I popped in an hour ago but you were asleep. We will come back soon after we have lunch.

[Friday, 2 May 2014 7:12:21 PM] Me: I am awake at moment

[Saturday, 3 May 2014 6:44:51 AM] Me: Woke up normal but had sweats and chills

[Saturday, 3 May 2014 9:48:59 AM] Kevin Harris :   Will come around in half hr or so.

[Saturday, 3 May 2014 6:33:11 PM] Me: Have shifted but still in High Dependency Unit slept for four hrs

[Saturday, 3 May 2014 6:35:58 PM] Kevin Harris :   Just spoke to dr but he didn't tell me you had moved! That's great hopefully a bit quieter there. Will be back there in an hour or so [

[Sunday, 4 May 2014 6:07:38 AM] Me: had good night much quieter

[Sunday, 4 May 2014 7:40:17 AM] Me: Seems I have sort of clear day, wondering if you could come early like 10am and help me do exercise's just for half hr and maybe after lunch same

[Sunday, 4 May 2014 7:42:33 AM] Kevin Harris :   Yes will do.

[Sunday, 4 May 2014 2:00:56 PM] Kevin Harris :   Donna on way walking probably nearly there b

[Monday, 5 May 2014 6:51:33 AM] Me: Had good night

[Monday, 5 May 2014 7:04:56 AM] Kevin Harris: Good to hear about night.

[Monday, 5 May 2014 9:53:47 AM] Me: Just been told rehab coming tomorrow regards sending me to St Margarete's hospital could go home first? told them to ring you

[Monday, 5 May 2014 5:40:43 PM] Me: Bring my wheelchair and walk stick please

[Tuesday, 6 May 2014 5:56:48 AM] Me: had good night but three huge sweats been up to toilet !!!!!! while they redid bed

[Tuesday, 6 May 2014 8:30:10 AM] Kevin Harris: Will be there about 9-30

[Tuesday, 6 May 2014 5:48:10 PM] Me: Chemo has been stopped as I swelled up

[Tuesday, 6 May 2014 6:35:14 PM] Me: can you come now please

[Tuesday, 6 May 2014 6:36:08 PM] Kevin Harris: Yes on way

[Wednesday, 7 May 2014 5:57:07 AM] Me: Up to midnight she changed the bed four times! Dry now amazing lets hope steroids work

[Wednesday, 7 May 2014 6:41:28 AM] Kevin Harris: Yes think steroids the best to keep under control. Hopefully they keep giving to you even if they don't give chemo.

[Wednesday, 7 May 2014 6:46:35 AM] Me: They told me I have a very big day and get sleep now will need donna from early like 9am i think

[Thursday, 8 May 2014 7:14:00 AM] Me: Had good night no chills just damp when woke at 5am slept all night feel ok

[Friday, 9 May 2014 6:51:47 AM] Me: A full night sleep no problems

[Friday, 9 May 2014 5:51:20 PM] Kevin Harris: Coming there soon.

[Saturday, 10 May 2014 6:18:10 AM] Me: Another good night

[Sunday, 11 May 2014 8:04:45 AM] Me: Reasonable night

[Sunday, 11 May 2014 3:01:48 PM] Me: Dr said having meeting here in morn with rehab don't know time?

[Sunday, 11 May 2014 6:21:12 PM] Kevin Harris :   We will visit there shortly

[Monday, 12 May 2014 8:01:48 AM] Me: Overnight ok except heartburn

[Monday, 12 May 2014 12:21:53 PM] Kevin Harris: How's things going there, heard from Dr or rehab people?

[Monday, 12 May 2014 6:57:46 PM] Me: No, hot here as need wet towel

[Monday, 12 May 2014 6:58:54 PM] Kevin Harris :   Just leaving work. Keep pushing button! Turn on fan

[Tuesday, 13 May 2014 8:13:08 AM] Me: Reasonable night but very uncomfortable they never took catheter out till 2am? Dr insisted Midnight. ok at moment

[Tuesday, 13 May 2014 8:16:21 AM] Me: Worried about good foot as is really ballooned they have no interest other than Chemo!

[Tuesday, 13 May 2014 8:40:39 AM] Kevin Harris :   I will talk to Dr about foot when I come in after lunch

[Tuesday, 13 May 2014 9:22:57 AM] Me: Its just fluid had salon on overnight now up showered now yet another chest xray then hope to get in wheelchair

[Wednesday, 14 May 2014 7:39:10 AM] Me: Night ok no fever

[Wednesday, 14 May 2014 7:40:36 AM] Kevin Harris: Good to hear. Rex will be there about 9-30

[Thursday, 15 May 2014 10:01:11 AM] Me: Ok overnight rex coming soon and have physio

[Thursday, 15 May 2014 11:50:21 AM] Me: Rehab both been both stress have to confirm where going live she says can install whatever in your house or need confirm gov house or what ever

[Friday, 16 May 2014 9:17:17 AM] Me: Good night slow start

[Friday, 16 May 2014 10:29:44 AM] Kevin Harris : Spoke to St Margaret's and they are happy with my place as discharge address, doesn't matter whether you end up going there or not. They won't take you with heartburn and swollen leg.

[Friday, 16 May 2014 11:56:51 AM] Me: thanks i think i need GP

[Tuesday, 20 May 2014 5:53:28 PM] Kevin Harris: Will see you tomorrow.

[Tuesday, 20 May 2014 5:57:38 PM] Me: Have meeting 10am with rehab re final details

[Tuesday, 20 May 2014 5:59:11 PM] Kevin Harris: That meeting is on Thursday so I will there, no problem.

[Tuesday, 20 May 2014 6:01:18 PM] Me: Doesn't appear so can you be there

[Tuesday, 20 May 2014 6:02:40 PM] Kevin Harris: Yes I will be there Thursday morning. I will come and see you tomorrow after work too

[Wednesday, 21 May 2014 3:39:26 PM] Me: i move between 10 and 11 in the morning no need to be here but can you come to night

[Wednesday, 21 May 2014 4:01:58 PM] Kevin Harris: Yes I have taken tomorrow off to see the Drs etc. not sure what time I get there hopefully before 7

[Wednesday, 21 May 2014 4:06:22 PM] Me: Not much point tomorrow they all geared pick me and go

[Wednesday, 21 May 2014 4:06:48 PM] Kevin Harris: Yes but want to see Drs and social worker and can't find time otherwise.

Insert: Arrived at Saint Margaret Hospital by Ambulance from the Queen Elizabeth Hospital.

[Friday, 23 May 2014 7:35:23 AM] Me: had a good night

[Friday, 23 May 2014 7:46:55 AM] Kevin Harris: Great was worried about the traffic noise but you will get used to it. Have a good morning with and hopefully get to look around a bit.

[Saturday, 24 May 2014 9:08:22 AM] Me: turned bed off at 2am hot some sleep at 4:30am was bascally flat other wise a good night. the list TV and areial and extension small radio jean shorts that small table out of van. sitting in sun

[Saturday, 24 May 2014 10:27:01 AM] Me: any dvds that might suit me

[Saturday, 24 May 2014 10:30:22 AM] Me: multi box

[Saturday, 24 May 2014 10:42:06 AM] Me: this radio now no go so the radio to find is about 300mmx 200mm new battery and power need batteries thanks

[Saturday, 24 May 2014 10:50:40 AM] Kevin Harris :   Ok got it all. Have few things to do at home then will go to storage place. Meeting guy at flat 2pm so might come and see you after that.

[Saturday, 24 May 2014 6:25:28 PM] Kevin Harris: Forgot to turn bed air pump back on! Hope nurse did for you.

[Sunday, 25 May 2014 7:54:57 AM] Me: thanks yesterday comfortable here feel much better knowing will have flat had good night

[Sunday, 25 May 2014 12:32:21 PM] Me: just eat complete plate Roast lamb mint sauce roast potatoe punkin collie!!!! yes need more lemonade too sorry on last bottle

[Sunday, 25 May 2014 12:37:44 PM] Kevin Harris : Bloody hell sounds great Sunday roast! We at semaphore having lunch then supermarket then will be there.

[Monday, 26 May 2014 10:09:29 AM] Me: Mellissa been suggests we go flat tomorrow about 3/4pm Doc been now QEH wants see me before frid as may change frid?

[Monday, 26 May 2014 10:10:28 AM] Me: tomorrow is her only avl day this week

[Monday, 26 May 2014 10:57:28 AM] Kevin Harris : Spoken to Melissa will confirm later this week. Dr going to call me back about visit to QEH

[Monday, 26 May 2014 11:45:02 AM] Me: dont worry radio today have radio on ipad/iph just done my washihg now in dryer!!!

[Monday, 26 May 2014 11:48:09 AM] Kevin Harris : Ok will see how I go. You've done washing!! May as well cook lunch too!

[Tuesday, 27 May 2014 9:20:51 AM] Me: night was ok

[Tuesday, 27 May 2014 9:26:54 AM] Kevin Good to hear night was good.

[Tuesday, 27 May 2014 4:51:35 PM] Me: everythink ok here dont worry coming tpnight

[Tuesday, 27 May 2014 7:50:48 PM] Kevin Harris : Hopefully you can read these. Will pop in tomorrow after work

[Thursday, 29 May 2014 3:44:59 PM] Me: appr QE 10.30am x2 ?? being picked up 10am are you able to get time off and meet me there they say an hr?

[Thursday, 29 May 2014 3:55:06 PM] Kevin): Yes can meet you there at 10-30. [Friday, 30 May 2014 2:18:00 PM] Kevin Ok. Has chemo started?

[Friday, 30 May 2014 7:56:10 PM] Me: new appt time frid 20th NE1b 11.30am

[Saturday, 31 May 2014 5:40:22 AM] Me: re radio I need a good small sterio for flat looked around and found one at harvey norman (sent email link) which will have remote no hurry

[Saturday, 31 May 2014 9:51:33 AM] Me: been awake since 3am

[Saturday, 31 May 2014 12:14:16 PM] Kevin Harris Will visit there in about an hour.

[Monday, 2 June 2014 8:04:16 AM] Me: New sterio great thanks have shifted to in window bed side

[Monday, 2 June 2014 1:24:40 PM] Kevin Harris the hospital arranging taxi for you and we will all meet there at unit at 3-45pm tomorrow.

[Tuesday, 3 June 2014 8:55:27 AM] Kevin Harris Has chemo nurse arrived yet to take chemo off?

[Tuesday, 3 June 2014 9:03:19 AM] Me: no

[Tuesday, 3 June 2014 9:04:24 AM] Kevin Harris   Ok hopefully soon. [Tuesday, 3 June 2014 12:01:22 PM] Me: Vinny coming 2pm . I will take my wheel chair in taxi and u can take after.

[Tuesday, 3 June 2014 2:59:49 PM] Kevin Harris Did nurse finish everything. What times taxi booked?

[Tuesday, 3 June 2014 3:02:52 PM] Me: chemo nurse finished gone got taxi 3.30pm

[Wednesday, 4 June 2014 7:59:03 AM] Me: flat looks good

[Thursday, 5 June 2014 12:51:51 PM] Me: I am very flat today been in bed all day giving me blood transf this afterernoon and another here tomorrow

[Thursday, 5 June 2014 12:52:40 PM] Kevin Harris ok blood will help get you back up a bit. Good that they do there. Buts it's all expected so just go with it and take 1 day at a time.

[Thursday, 5 June 2014 3:11:17 PM] Me: temp went up with blood so stopped jt its coming down now and going start again

[Thursday, 5 June 2014 3:37:33 PM] Kevin Harris How's temperature? Getting blood still?

[Friday, 6 June 2014 7:01:17 AM] Me: another lot of blood today feel ok .

[Friday, 6 June 2014 7:07:00 AM] Kevin Harris Good that transfusions help. Called nurse last night about blood during weekend if needed and she said you were asleep.

[Friday, 6 June 2014 2:13:44 PM] Kevin Harris Feeling ok, did you get another lot of blood?

[Friday, 6 June 2014 2:18:53 PM] Me: no they canceled blood feel ok been in bed ad cold got no food or cash vend wont take notes stock up Sunday

[Friday, 6 June 2014 5:36:24 PM] Kevin Harris will drop in there about 9-30am. [

[Saturday, 7 June 2014 6:50:58 AM] Me: woke early washing on 6am coffee from machine feeling ok. you said you may come around 9:30am

[Sunday, 8 June 2014 10:06:16 AM] Kevin Harris Be there 10 mins

[Monday, 9 June 2014 7:13:43 AM] Me: can only go out on weekends i am ok thanks

[Monday, 9 June 2014 10:34:00 AM] Kevin Ok, we could maybe ask if you could come out in mid afternoon for an hour after Physio etc finished.

[Monday, 9 June 2014 10:50:14 AM] Me: havnt had xshower not much sting in me today just had bread olive oil bit crook gut finally got laptop updated and on wifi very tired think just sleep today.

[Monday, 9 June 2014 10:55:20 AM] Kevin Ok that's fine though, just rest. Not sure when last blood test was but maybe ask them to do one today. You may need unit of blood.

[Monday, 9 June 2014 10:57:38 AM] Me: no one here knows what they doing all standins

[Monday, 9 June 2014 11:01:41 AM] Kevin Harris Ok, will make sure tests get done tomorrow so your system doesn't get too low.

[Monday, 9 June 2014 11:03:10 AM] Me well the head nurse just walked in to take blood there u go

[Tuesday, 10 June 2014 6:37:51 AM] Me: Consultant Drs here this morning between 9 and 10:30 for Prothesis going to ask how long it takes need to get idea how much longer here so can plan my life.Feeling better today except my guts

[Tuesday, 10 June 2014 10:02:02 AM] Me: drs been next week go to prospect for cast then they make it then have to learn to walk so here for up to another 4 weeks or so

[Tuesday, 10 June 2014 10:35:17 AM] Kevin Harris Ok good to hear your feeling ok except stomach and that time frame for walking etc sounds about right I guess.

[Tuesday, 10 June 2014 12:51:13 PM] Me: ok

[Wednesday, 11 June 2014 11:19:29 AM] Kevin Harris Ok sounds good , will arrange a time to get it done with them.

[Wednesday, 11 June 2014 2:17:46 PM] Me: having more blood this afternoon

[Wednesday, 11 June 2014 2:27:10 PM] Kevin Harris: Not too much, that's stuffs expensive!

[Thursday, 12 June 2014 7:32:12 AM] Kevin Harris Feel better after some new blood? Will drop in after work, so let me know if anything you need me to bring.

[Thursday, 12 June 2014 8:29:44 AM] Me: A bit flat today will let you know if need anything

[Friday, 13 June 2014 10:04:43 AM] Me: have permission from dr who just came out of the blue for sat dont be late as only have 10 to 2

[Friday, 13 June 2014 10:16:56 AM] Kevin Harris): Better hope weather a lot better than today

[Saturday, 14 June 2014 9:26:03 AM] Me: when arive in car park turn rightt and back around so i get in op side to hosp

[Saturday, 14 June 2014 6:39:56 PM] Me: Thanks today was great went to sleep when came home size 14 perfect i feel helpess i just wish i could do more.

[Sunday, 15 June 2014 2:15:31 PM] Me: I will be getting out of here frid i am not giving them an option I am not laying around here boxed in laying in bed for maybe half hr physio each day its rediculouse At home i have proved i can manage and i will get more exercise is which they say i need!

I will be telling physio tomorrow and the doctor here and will dicuss with consultant on tues!!

[Monday, 16 June 2014 7:33:44 AM] Me: what if i can get out of here wed?? sooner better at $55/day do you think can get flat wed?

I just need a breakthrough in this life

[Monday, 16 June 2014 3:46:52 PM] Me: just walked on two legs no problem felt natural using a mockup leg physio says i can do physio at QEH

[Monday, 16 June 2014 4:03:25 PM] Kevin Harris (That's great news, welcome back to two legs for a little bit! So chemo and Physio can both be done at QEH as outpatient.

[Monday, 16 June 2014 4:14:51 PM] Me: physio has no problem with me leaving here!! will talk consultant in morning but where do i go. I wonder if i explain situation to the Social worker here if he can sort?

[Monday, 16 June 2014 8:59:04 PM] Kevin Harris Platform finished, hopefully fits, or else will use saw! Have reworked calc and yes need 800x2100 for ramp. Before I had it lying opposite way

[Monday, 16 June 2014 9:06:10 PM] Me: thanks for doing deck.

[Tuesday, 17 June 2014 8:14:58 AM] Me: had my first fall about 3am sat on side of bed and stretched out for bottle whips slipped happened fast my shoulder crashed into unit which took most of fall and ended on floor . took a bit to get back up. i am ok

[Tuesday, 17 June 2014 8:19:10 AM] Kevin Harris Bloody hell, guess falls are always going to happen an it gives you some sense of what's possible and not possible to do at this stage. Go easy, no more injuries!

[Tuesday, 17 June 2014 10:16:56 AM] Kevin Harris (+Ok just heard and If you are discharged and all ok you can move there on Friday ! I'm having time off Friday to see dr etc so can help move too.

[Tuesday, 17 June 2014 10:17:57 AM] Me: They are having meeting shortly to confirm my discharge not sure from when but going for stump fitting tomorrow!!!!

[Tuesday, 17 June 2014 10:23:09 AM] Kevin Harris Yes chemo and dr Friday. Pls leave discharge until Friday, I can't have time off thurs and Friday.

[Tuesday, 17 June 2014 10:25:42 AM] Me: ok see what i can do

[Tuesday, 17 June 2014 11:19:57 AM] Me: what time is apt frid Qe??

[Tuesday, 17 June 2014 11:26:32 AM] Kevin Harris It's at 11-30am.

[Tuesday, 17 June 2014 7:39:07 PM] Me: could you ask if i can take it from thurs as gail is coming on thurs she could shift all imy gear from here plus go supermarket stock up meat food etc sort flat need fridge freezer what do you think?

[Tuesday, 17 June 2014 8:46:16 PM] Kevin Harris : given go ahead for Thursday. The rail and shower hose was done today. Your wheel chair and shower chair being delivered there Friday. new leg on order, things are looking up!!

[Wednesday, 18 June 2014 7:15:36 AM] Kevin Harris Friday the priority is Dr and day of chemo. Also need to be at house for Dom care dropping off gear. Still need to do ramp.

[Wednesday, 18 June 2014 7:22:51 AM] Me: I want a car asap i need my freedom

[Wednesday, 18 June 2014 10:21:12 AM] Kevin Harris Pls wait until we see dr on Friday and discuss teet many etc with him before making decisions on buying a car. Chemo intake and side effects have priority over anything else.

[Wednesday, 18 June 2014 11:57:43 AM] Me: i am being discharged at 10am frid having instructions and medication explained then they send me via access taxie to Qe for 11 am apt I am at place getting cast of stump. I will be able to do things so it takes the load off you and will be able to come here etc for fittings without you like apt here next tues because i will have my own car

[Wednesday, 18 June 2014 4:35:32 PM] Me: Got plastered!!! measured other leg and foot go back tues (mile end) she called it a fitting dont know if she means just the part that slips on or the whole thing??

[Thursday, 19 June 2014 2:36:23 PM] Me: have new wheel chair!!! light and smooth !!!

[Thursday, 19 June 2014 4:42:59 PM] Kevin Harris Good to hear about wheel chair hopefully easy to manage in/out car

[Thursday, 19 June 2014 8:03:36 PM] Kevin Harris Will see you at 10-30 at QEH

[Thursday, 19 June 2014 8:06:52 PM] Me: ok thanks

Going to be a long day I recon. just wish i could help with ramp.

[Friday, 20 June 2014 9:42:37 AM] Me: time changed taxie now booked 10:40am so will be late. Remind me update address at reception

[Friday, 20 June 2014 9:49:08 AM] Kevin Harris Ok will see you there at 11-00. Going to drop off platform then will go get ply and drop that back. [Friday, 20 June 2014 9:49:12 AM] Kevin Harris (Do you have your drivers license as I don't think here?

[Friday, 20 June 2014 9:50:13 AM] Me: yes i have it

[Friday, 20 June 2014 9:52:03 AM] Me: before you get ply out get some metle strip or hinges to fix ramp each side to deck

Insert: Arrived at the Queen Elizabeth Hospital from Saint Margaret Hospital by Access Cab.

[Friday, 20 June 2014 11:02:26 AM] Me: here but out at ambulance

[Friday, 20 June 2014 11:01:44 AM] Kevin Harris Ok will walk that way outside on street

[Friday, 20 June 2014 11:04:34 AM] Me: l amat transport

Insert: After meeting my son at the hospital I visited the Cancer Clinic for the start of the third round of Chemo I was then formally released from Hospital and went home to my flat to live my life and undergo the remainder of my treatment.

End of Text Transcripts

End of this Publication

Rev 01.04.2018